THE COVID-19 CRISIS

Since its emergence in early 2020, the COVID-19 crisis has affected every part of the world. Well beyond its health effects, the pandemic has wrought major changes in people's everyday lives as they confront restrictions imposed by physical distancing and consequences such as loss of work, working or learning from home and reduced contact with family and friends.

This edited collection covers a diverse range of experiences, practices and representations across international contexts and cultures (UK, Europe, North America, South Africa, Australia and New Zealand). Together, these contributions offer a rich account of COVID society. They provide snapshots of what life was like for people in a variety of situations and locations living through the first months of the novel coronavirus crisis, including discussion not only of health-related experiences but also the impact on family, work, social life and leisure activities. The socio-material dimensions of quotidian practices are highlighted: death rituals, dating apps, online musical performances, fitness and exercise practices, the role of windows, healthcare work, parenting children learning at home, moving in public space as a blind person and many more diverse topics are explored. In doing so, the authors surface the feelings of strangeness and challenges to norms of practice that were part of many people's experiences, highlighting the profound affective responses that accompanied the disruption to usual cultural forms of sociality and ritual in the wake of the COVID outbreak and restrictions on movement. The authors show how social relationships and social institutions were suspended, re-invented or transformed while social differences were brought to the fore.

At the macro level, the book includes localised and comparative analyses of political, health system and policy responses to the pandemic, and highlights the differences in representations and experiences of very different social groups, including people with disabilities, LGBTQI people, Dutch Muslim parents, healthcare workers in France and Australia, young adults living in northern Italy, performing artists and their audiences, exercisers in Australia and New Zealand, the Latin cultures of Spain and Italy, Asian-Americans and older people in Australia. This volume will appeal to undergraduates and postgraduates in sociology, cultural and media studies, medical humanities, anthropology, political science and cultural geography.

Deborah Lupton is SHARP Professor in the Centre for Social Research in Health and the Social Policy Research Centre at the University of New South Wales (UNSW) Sydney, Australia, leading the Vitalities Lab and the UNSW Node of the Australian Research Council Centre of Excellence for Automated Decision-Making + Society.

Karen Willis is Professor, School of Allied Health, Human Services and Sport, La Trobe University, Melbourne, Australia, and Honorary Professor, Division of Critical Care and Investigative Services, Royal Melbourne Hospital.

THE COVID-19 CRISIS

Social Perspectives

Edited by Deborah Lupton and Karen Willis

Routledge
Taylor & Francis Group
LONDON AND NEW YORK

First published 2021
by Routledge
2 Park Square, Milton Park, Abingdon, Oxon OX14 4RN

and by Routledge
52 Vanderbilt Avenue, New York, NY 10017

Routledge is an imprint of the Taylor & Francis Group, an informa business

British Library Cataloguing-in-Publication Data
A catalogue record for this book is available from the British Library

Library of Congress Cataloging-in-Publication Data
Names: Lupton, Deborah, editor. | Willis, Karen, 1960- editor.
Title: The COVID-19 crisis : social perspectives / edited by Deborah Lupton and Karen Willis.
Description: Abingdon, Oxon ; New York, NY : Routledge, 2021. | Includes bibliographical references and index.
Identifiers: LCCN 2020052383 (print) | LCCN 2020052384 (ebook) | ISBN 9780367628956 (hardback) | ISBN 9780367628987 (paperback) | ISBN 9781003111344 (ebook)
Subjects: LCSH: COVID-19 (Disease)--Social aspects. | Public health--Social aspects. | Epidemics--Social aspects.
Classification: LCC RA644.C67 C6833 2021 (print) | LCC RA644.C67 (ebook) | DDC 362.1962/414--dc23
LC record available at https://lccn.loc.gov/2020052383
LC ebook record available at https://lccn.loc.gov/2020052384

ISBN: 978-0-367-62895-6 (hbk)
ISBN: 978-0-367-62898-7 (pbk)
ISBN: 978-1-003-11134-4 (ebk)

Typeset in Bembo
by Taylor & Francis Books

CONTENTS

PART V
Marginalisation and discrimination 181

ILLUSTRATIONS

Figures

Table

CONTRIBUTORS

Susan Banks is a research fellow in the Tasmanian Policy Exchange, University of Tasmania, Australia, and a chief investigator in the Preventing Elder Abuse in Tasmania (PEAT) research group.

Julie Brice is a doctoral student in Te Huataki Waiora/School of Health at Te Whare Wānanga o Waikato/University of Waikato, Aotearoa/New Zealand.

Nicola Burns is a lecturer in disability studies in the Department of Sociology at the University of Glasgow, UK, and is co-investigator on the Wellcome Trust funded project 'Doctors within Borders: Networking Initiative on Mobile Populations in Contemporary Health Systems' (2019–2021).

Marianne Clark is a postdoctoral research fellow in the Vitalities Lab, Centre for Social Research in Health and Social Policy Research Centre, UNSW Sydney, Australia.

Peta S. Cook is a senior lecturer of sociology and course coordinator (ageing studies and services) at the Wicking Dementia Centre, University of Tasmania, Australia, and conducts research on ageing, age-inclusive environments, and health and wellbeing.

Cassie Curryer (PhD sociology and anthropology) is a postdoctoral research fellow at the University of Newcastle, Australia, where her research explores the nexus between public health, gender, housing, and social policy systems.

Christopher Dietzel is a PhD candidate at McGill University, Tiohtiá:ke/Montreal, Canada, where his research explores sexuality, gender, violence, safety and digital media technologies.

Stefanie Duguay is an assistant professor in the Department of Communication Studies at Concordia University in Tiohtiá:ke/Montreal, Canada, where her research focuses on the intersection of sexual identity, gender, and digital media technologies.

Jordi Farré is senior lecturer in journalism and communication at Rovira i Virgili University, Spain, leading the Asterisc Communication Research Group, where she conducts research on risk and health communication, organisational and media logic.

Karolina Follis is a senior lecturer in the Department of Politics, Philosophy and Religion at Lancaster University, UK, leading the Wellcome Trust-funded project 'Doctors within Borders: Networking Initiative on Mobile Populations in Contemporary Health Systems' (2019–2021).

Luca Follis is senior lecturer in law and society at Lancaster University Law School, UK, and co-investigator on the Wellcome Trust-funded project 'Doctors within Borders: Networking Initiative on Mobile Populations in Contemporary Health Systems' (2019–2021).

Gaëtan Gentile is university professor, chair of the Department of General Practice at Aix-Marseille-University, France, and research associate at the Institut des Neurosciences des Systemes (INSERM/AMU).

Anne M. Harris is professor, Australian Research Council Future Fellow and RMIT Vice Chancellor's Senior Research Fellow, RMIT University, Melbourne, Australia. She is the director of the Creative Agency Lab at RMIT.

Anna Hickey-Moody is professor of media and communication, Australian Research Council Future Fellow and RMIT Vice Chancellor's Senior Research Fellow, RMIT University, Melbourne, Australia. She is a visiting professor in sociology at Goldsmiths, University of London, UK, and treasurer of the Australian Sociological Association.

Jack Lam is a research fellow at the University of Queensland Institute for Social Science Research and the ARC Centre of Excellence for Children and Families over the Life Course, Brisbane, Australia, and conducts research in families, health and ageing.

Linda Lombi is senior researcher at the Università Cattolica del Sacro Cuore, Milan, Italy. Her research focuses on health sociology, participatory medicine, patient engagement and digital health.

Sakina Loukili is a PhD candidate at the Meertens Institute and VU University, Amsterdam, the Netherlands. Her research focuses on social media, religion, (national) identity and politics.

Heidi Lourens is a senior lecturer in the Department of Psychology, University of Johannesburg, South Africa.

Alessandro Lovari is assistant professor of sociology of communication at the Department of Political and Social Sciences, University of Cagliari, Italy. His research focuses on public sector communication, social media and health communication.

Deborah Lupton is SHARP Professor in the Centre for Social Research in Health and the Social Policy Research Centre at the University of New South Wales (UNSW) Sydney, Australia, leading the Vitalities Lab and the UNSW Node of the Australian Research Council Centre of Excellence for Automated Decision-Making + Society.

Romain Lutaud is general practitioner (MD), PhD candidate in public health and social sciences, and research fellow and lecturer at the Department of General Practice, Aix-Marseille University, France. His research broaches the issues of care pathways in situations of uncertainty and scientific controversy.

Annetta H. Mallon is an honorary adjunct with Western Sydney University specialising in end of life and is a qualitative social researcher in the arenas of non-medical end of life work and roles.

Antonio Maturo is professor of medical sociology at Bologna University, Italy. He is also the chair of the PhD programme in sociology and social research.

Veronica Moretti is a research fellow at Bologna University, Italy. Her research interests focus on digital health, STS and surveillance theories.

Janine Morley is researcher at Lancaster University, UK, where she works on the 'Doctors within Borders: Networking Initiative on Mobile Populations in Contemporary Health Systems' project (2019–2021).

Olimpia Mosteanu is a PhD in sociology, currently working as a senior researcher at Social Life in London, UK. Her research interests are located at the intersection of the fields of housing and health.

Jo Murphy-Lawless is a research fellow in the Centre for Health Evaluation, Methodology Research and Evidence Synthesis, NUI Galway, Ireland.

Paul Mutsaers is assistant professor at the Department of Anthropology and Development Studies of Radboud University, the Netherlands, and affiliated to Border Criminologies, University of Oxford, Faculty of Law, UK.

David Myles is affiliate professor in sexology at the Université du Québec à Montréal and a postdoctoral fellow at the Institute for Gender, Sexuality and Feminist Studies, McGill University, Canada.

Barbara Barbosa Neves is senior lecturer in sociology at Monash University, Melbourne, Australia.

Lucy Nicholas is associate professor in sociology and genders and sexualities, and director of genders and sexualities research at Western Sydney University, Australia.

Maho Omori is a research fellow at the School of Social Sciences (sociology), Monash University, Melbourne, Australia, and conducts research in ageing, health and residential aged care.

Alex Schenkels is a PhD candidate at the Department of Culture Studies of Tilburg University and lecturer at the School of Pedagogical Studies of Fontys University of Applied Sciences, the Netherlands.

Anna Sendra is a postdoctoral fellow at the Department of Communication of University of Ottawa, Canada, and a member of the ASTERISC Communication Research Group of Universitat Rovira i Virgili, Spain. Her research focuses on health communication, chronic diseases, and digital health.

Natasha Smallwood is a consultant respiratory physician at the Royal Melbourne Hospital and principal research fellow (associate professor) in the Department of Medicine at the University of Melbourne, Australia. She leads a programme of research in advanced lung disease, but also has research interests in healthcare worker wellbeing and health leadership.

Ryan Thorneycroft is lecturer in criminology in the School of Social Sciences at Western Sydney University, Australia.

Holly Thorpe is professor of sport and physical cultural studies in Te Huataki Waiora School of Health, University of Waikato, New Zealand.

Pierre Verger, MD, is an epidemiologist and director of the regional health observatory Provence-Alpes-Cote d'Azur (ORS PACA). His research interests focus on the practices and attitudes of family physicians, particularly towards vaccination.

Jeremy K. Ward is a sociologist and postdoctoral fellow at the CNRS (French National Centre for Scientific Research) in the Groupe d'étude des méthodes de l'analyse sociologique de la Sorbonne. His research broaches the issues of lay attitudes to science and sociotechnical controversies. Most of his work has dealt with vaccine hesitancy and public debates over vaccination.

Marissa Willcox is a PhD candidate in the School of Media and Communication at RMIT University in Melbourne, Australia. Her research looks at gender and sexuality in art practice online and she also works as a project manager on the ARC funded 'Interfaith Childhoods' project.

Karen Willis is Professor, School of Allied Health, Human Services and Sport, La Trobe University, Melbourne, Australia, and Honorary Professor, Division of Critical Care and Investigative Services, Royal Melbourne Hospital.

Aggie J. Yellow Horse is an assistant professor in Asian Pacific American studies in the School of Social Transformation at Arizona State University, USA.

ACKNOWLEDGEMENTS

The impetus for this book came from the overwhelming response to our call for submissions for a special section of *Health Sociology Review* (volume 29, issue 2, 2020). We wish to thank *Health Sociology Review* for their continuing support of this project. We also acknowledge the support of the Centre for Social Research in Health and the Social Policy Research Centre, UNSW Sydney, and the School of Allied Health, Human Services and Sport, La Trobe University. We thank the Social Research Assistance Platform, La Trobe University, for providing funding for editorial assistance, and Jane Emery for providing this assistance with the final draft.

PART I
Introduction

1

COVID SOCIETY

Introduction to the book

Deborah Lupton and Karen Willis

Introduction

In the early 1990s, the English translation of the German sociologist Ulrich Beck's book *Risk Society: Towards a New Modernity* (Beck, 1992) introduced the concept of 'risk society' to sociologists and risk theorists internationally. Beck argued that processes of industrialisation and globalisation had led to a way of thinking in which people had become highly sensitised to the risks that had proliferated as an outcome of modernisation. His 'risk society' was a world in which ideas and understandings about selfhood, social relations and social institutions were increasingly framed through the lens of risk, associated with an intensifying sense of threat, danger and uncertainty and a desire to systematically manage these threats and insecurities. In an historical and geographical context in which environmental disasters (including the 1986 Chernobyl nuclear power plant disaster) dominated the risk landscape, Beck's work focused on the hazards and uncertainties of pollution and climate change. He defined the 'risks of modernisation' as 'irreversible threats to the life of plants, animals, and human beings' (Beck, 1992: 13).

Beck's risk society thesis sparked an outpouring of sociological work in the 1990s and early 2000s, in which social theory and empirical studies sought to identify how risks were generated, understood and managed as social processes (Lupton, 2013). In recent years, risk theory has lost much of its prominence – overtaken by other 'turns' in social theory and other preoccupations by social researchers. However, the COVID-19 crisis has brought social responses to risk into renewed prominence. Almost three decades after the publication of *Risk Society*, it could be argued that we are now living in a global 'COVID society'. The emergence and rapid spread of the COVID-19 pandemic from the early months of 2020 has preoccupied public discourse and news media reporting and has sparked upheavals worldwide.

According to the World Health Organization (WHO), the first cases of an atypical viral pneumonia from an unknown cause was reported in a media statement by officials in Wuhan, China on the last day of 2019 (World Health Organization, 2020). WHO issued its first Disease Outbreak News report about these cases on 5 January 2020 and reported that the Chinese authorities had confirmed that the pathogen was a novel coronavirus. China reported the first death on 11 January and the first case outside China was reported by Thailand on 13 January. On 21 January, the possibility of human-to-human transmission was confirmed by WHO and the USA reported its first case of COVID. The first cases in Europe were reported by French authorities on 24 January. WHO declared a public health emergency of international concern on 30 January and on 11 February announced that the novel coronavirus would be named SARS-CoV-2 and the disease it caused as COVID-19 (a contraction of 'coronavirus disease 2019'). WHO declared that COVID-19 had reached pandemic status on 11 March, meaning that the epidemic had spread globally, crossing international borders and simultaneously affecting very large numbers of people in different parts of the world. At this point, Europe (and particularly Italy and Spain) had become the epicentre of the crisis. The UK, USA, Brazil and India were later to become the epicentres. By the end of June 2020, 10 million cases of infection with SARS-CoV-2 had been recorded globally, having doubled within six weeks, with over half a million confirmed deaths from COVID-19 (Du and Cortez, 2020).

No end is yet in sight for the pandemic, with global numbers continuing to rise, and many countries experiencing new surges of infections. The coronavirus has proven to be difficult to contain, once strict lockdown conditions are loosened. Greater tourist movements across national borders in the northern summer of 2020, for example, generated new surges of infection in countries such as Spain, Italy and France, while Australia's second largest city, Melbourne, went into a second lockdown in July 2020 after quarantine measures for incoming travellers from overseas were badly mismanaged. By the end of September 2020, the grim global tally of over 1 million deaths from COVID-19 had been confirmed, from over 33 million confirmed cases. The USA was still the country with the highest COVID cases and deaths, but India was rapidly catching up, with Brazil and Russia following closely behind. The problems of those experiencing 'long COVID' illness were beginning to be documented, demonstrating that COVID-19 for some people was a long-lasting health problem (Mahase, 2020).

The COVID pandemic is far more than a massive global health problem – it is a crisis on every level: social, cultural, environmental and economic. As a zoonotic disease (originating in animals and transferring to humans), COVID-19 is a product of human-environment relationships (Braidotti, 2020): even to the point that some commentators have argued that the coronavirus is the planet's revenge on humans for the damage it has sustained at our hands (Searle and Turnbull, 2020). However, the pandemic's effects reach well beyond these relationships. Few areas of everyday life have been left unchanged in the wake of the emergence of this new infectious disease. The COVID crisis is a complex and ever-thickening entanglement of people with other living things, place, space, objects, time, discourse and culture.

Social impacts of COVID-19

When the pandemic began to erupt globally, it soon became evident that detailed and situated social research was vital to understanding how the crisis was affecting people across the world. Sociologists have been interested in the sociocultural and political dimensions of epidemics and pandemics for some time, pointing out how fear, moralism, blame and Othering are often major societal responses (Dingwall et al., 2013; Strong, 1990; van Loon, 2005; Bjørkdahl and Carlsen, 2019). In April 2020, Geoffrey Pleyers (2020), the vice president of research for the International Sociological Association, published what he called 'a plea for global sociology in times of the coronavirus'. Pleyers noted that given the crisis had affected all dimensions of society – well beyond the health implications – responses to COVID required expertise in social research just as much as medical and public health expertise. He argued further that as the pandemic is a global phenomenon, a global perspective is required in addition to nation-based social research, so that researchers can learn from other countries' experiences.

Political responses were crucial to how well nations fared in the first phase of the pandemic (Afsahi et al., 2020; Gugushvili et al., 2020). In what has been described as 'biopolitical nationalism' (de Kloet et al., 2020), many governments implemented strict controls over citizens' movements and imposed surveillance and policing measures to enforce them. Nation-states retreated into themselves, erecting *cordons sanitaire* that in some cases segregated parts of cities as well imposing internal as well as international border controls in the attempt to control and contain the movements of human bodies infected with coronavirus (Afsahi et al., 2020). Citizens went through very different experiences of the COVID crisis based on how their governments and health officials reacted. Nations with liberal or populist leaders who failed to respond early enough with physical distancing measures, such as in the UK (Scambler, 2020), USA (Rocco et al., 2020; Thomson, 2020) and Brazil (Malta et al., 2020) floundered, recording far higher numbers of COVID infections and deaths (Gugushvili et al., 2020). Those countries where interventions were established earlier and with more extensive lockdown restrictions and border control measures, such as Taiwan, New Zealand, Vietnam, Australia, South Korea and Singapore, managed the spread of the pandemic much more successfully during its initial stages (Dalglish, 2020; Afsahi et al., 2020). There remains debate about countries such as Sweden, where the policy approach has been around 'living with' the virus and gaining 'herd immunity' (Pierre, 2020). All policy approaches have caused much debate about economic versus health outcomes – whether the longer term costs to societies of restrictions and lockdowns (caused by shutting down much economic activity) are outweighed by the health benefits in terms of reduced mortality, morbidity, and pressure on health systems.

Enforced quarantine, physical isolation, confinement to home, border closures, shutdowns of business, workplaces, schools and universities instituted in initial government responses to containing the spread of the virus have affected national economies, freedom of movement, familial and social relationships and mental wellbeing. Concepts of risk, uncertainty and trust suddenly had to be reassessed and confronted (Brown, 2020). It was obvious from the early months of the global spread of the coronavirus that while everyone was at risk from contracting the infection, in most countries some social groups were more at risk than others (Afsahi et al., 2020). These included groups that were already experiencing high levels of socioeconomic disadvantage, marginalisation and low access to health services, such as people with disabilities in Singapore and Australia (Goggin and Ellis, 2020), Indigenous Australians (Markham and Smith, 2020), Roma people in Europe (Matache and Bhabha, 2020), Black, Asian and minority ethnic groups in the UK (Bhatia, 2020), low caste and Muslim people in India (Rahman, 2020), Black Americans (Egede and Walker, 2020), Asian Americans (Roberto et al., 2020) and vulnerable and marginalised groups in Sweden, such as older people, immigrants and prisoners (Rambaree and Nässén, 2020). Gendered inequalities have also been exacerbated due to restrictions requiring working and learning from home. In many countries, women's opportunities to engage in paid employment have been severely affected by caring responsibilities as they were forced to juggle working from home with supervising their children's learning when schools were closed (Craig, 2020; Bahn et al., 2020; Al-Ali, 2020). Incidents of family violence have also escalated, with women finding it more difficult to seek help as they are forced to spend more time in the home with their abuser (Williamson et al., 2020).

To avoid infection – or infecting others – people were required to take up new social behaviours, such as more frequent handwashing, maintaining a physical distance from others outside their households, staying at home as much as possible, wearing face masks, relinquishing their usual leisure pursuits and avoiding gathering in groups with family members, friends or work colleagues. As Dahiya (2020) observed, 'The lived experience of COVID-19 forcibly returns us to our bodies'. People were forced to confront the nature of embodiment and interembodiment with others, and the risks that previously benign physical encounters with not only strangers but close family members and friends could bring. New forms of sociality and intimacy had to be developed to allow people to engage with others in times of physical distancing: often involving greater use of digital media such as texting and video-calling (Nguyen et al., 2020; Watson et al., 2020). A plethora of digital tools were also created to help manage and monitor the spread of coronavirus, including contact tracing apps, dashboards of COVID metrics and wearable devices to keep track of people under isolation orders (Everts, 2020; Meijer et al., 2020). These measures have raised privacy concerns in relation to how people's personal information is being used (Kitchin, 2020). However, other commentators have highlighted the deleterious effects of the opposite problem. 'Data invisibility' can adversely affect those (the 'data poor') whose experiences and health status are not recorded in official statistics and whose plight is therefore unrecognised (Milan and Treré, 2020).

The news media have played a crucial role in publicising information about COVID, including providing regular updates about infection and death rates globally and regionally and disseminating details about how publics can best protect themselves and others from coronavirus. There have been notable lapses, however, with concerns about the 'infodemic' (Orso et al., 2020) of mis-information and deliberate lies that have been spread on news and social media sites (Meese et al., 2020; Baker et al., 2020; Rodrigues and Xu, 2020). News coverage has also contributed to racism and the othering of social groups. Due to the Chinese origins of the first reported cases of COVID, racist statements and abuse were directed at Chinese people in everyday life and news media reporting in many countries, including Japan (Shimizu, 2020), Chile (Chan and Montt Strabucchi, 2020), the UK (Pang, 2020), the USA (Roberto et al., 2020) and India (Haokip, 2020).

This book

We are both sociologists who have specialised in researching health and medical topics throughout our careers. From early in the emergence and spread of the COVID-19 pandemic, we quickly recognised the importance of social researchers beginning to document the transformations in everyday life across the globe that COVID had begun to engender. At the end of March 2020, Deborah published an outline of what she described as an initial agenda for social research about COVID and post-COVID worlds (Lupton, 2020a) and sent out a call for contributions for a special section of *Health Sociology Review* she guest edited on sociology and COVID-19. This special section was published in July 2020 (Lupton, 2020b). Many excellent abstracts were submitted for consideration. As one of the chief editors of *Health Sociology Review*, Karen worked with Deborah to select the abstracts to go forward for full submission. The authors of other highly ranked abstracts were invited to contribute to an edited volume, and we were delighted to receive an enthusiastic response. Their contributions comprise the chapters in this book, providing insights into the social dimensions of COVID in Australia, France, Italy, Ireland, New Zealand, Spain, South Africa, the Netherlands, the UK, Canada and the USA.

All chapters were conceived, written, submitted, revised and finalised within seven months of the WHO's declaration of the pandemic: a period of rapid spread and sudden changes in everyday life as nations struggled to contain the infection. Given the continuing effects of the COVID crisis, with many countries experiencing resurgences and still struggling to find the best way to deal with the coronavirus as well as its related socioeconomic effects, the book stands as a way of documenting this initial period. It is divided into topical sections. Immediately following this chapter in Part I ('Introduction') is Deborah Lupton's overview of sociocultural perspectives on contagion in the literature published prior to the COVID outbreak (Chapter 2). Lupton's chapter is designed to establish a firm context for the COVID-focused chapters that follow. The perspectives offered by social histories, political economy perspectives, social constructionism, Foucauldian theory, risk theory, postcolonial and sociomaterial approaches are explained and examples of research using these approaches are provided.

In Part II ('Space, the Body and Mobilities'), the analysis by Nicola Burns, Luca Follis, Karolina Follis and Janine Morley (Chapter 3) focuses on the UK government's response to COVID, emphasising the multi-scalar effects of state intervention and the implications for different groups in society. Some of these inequalities cohered around mobilities: those who were allowed out of their homes and expected to move in public spaces to perform essential duties, and those who were considered vulnerable or non-essential and expected to dramatically reduce their movements.

In Chapter 4, Holly Thorpe, Julie Briggs and Marianne Clark also discuss aspects of embodiment and movement. Engaging with poetic representations of experience, their chapter critically explores new questions about the risks of physically active human bodies and the 'trails' of contagion that they may disperse in and through the ebbs and flows of the natural (air, wind) and built (gym and fitness studios) environment. In so doing, they offer a critical and creative commentary on the new noticings of bodily boundaries in times of pandemic, where every puffing, panting individual encountered moving through space was a source of possible contagion via their bodily fluids and excretions.

Olimpia Mosteanu's (Chapter 5) chapter also directs attention to the socio-materialities of people's bodies with the built environment, with a focus on the ways that windows operated as parts of human-home assemblages during the COVID lockdown period in London. Drawing on a series of photographs she had taken, Mosteanu explores some of the ways in which windows not only mediate our interactions with the world around us but also actively participate in our everyday lives in a time at which many people are feeling confined, isolated and restless.

In recounting her experiences as a person living with visual impairment, Heidi Lourens (Chapter 6) demonstrates how it feels to be living with COVID risk and treated as a vulnerable person – or worse, objectified as less than human. She highlights the ways in which touch is used to help people with visual impairment and how touch has become suffused with particular risk of contagion. Lourens argues for a relational ethics of care that can encompass mutual respect and recognition of these feelings and needs for both people living with disabilities and those who are not: all of whom are faced with managing the risks of contagion, but in different ways.

Part III ('Intimacies, Socialities and Connections') begins with an analysis of how dating app companies participated in disseminating COVID health messages. David Myles, Stefanie Duguay and Christopher Dietzel (Chapter 7) show how these companies rapidly re-positioned their key strategies and messages to deal with challenges to their user base and business model. A re-invented concept, 'dating while distancing', sought to demonstrate the utility of such apps for a new relationships paradigm in which the old ways of connecting and meeting could no longer take place due to physical distancing restrictions.

In Chapter 8, drawing on interviews with young northern Italians, Veronica Moretti and Antonio Maturo show how perceptions of time, space and domestic habits changed during this period of immense disruption to everyday routines and social encounters. Moretti and Maturo describe how for young professionals, being forced to stay at home was a cognitively ambiguous situation, in which their normal lives were in suspension.

Ryan Thorneycroft and Lucy Nicholas (Chapter 9) then interrogate sexual practices occurring during COVID-19 to imagine alternative (crip and queer) futures. They argue that understanding our moment through what they characterise as 'crip/queer times' provides the opportunity to open up new sexual cultures and to diversify the range of practices and pleasures to *all* people. In the place of queer casual sex, Thorneycroft and Nicholas introduce forms of (crip/queer) isolation sex as an efficacious and ethical alternative, identifying new forms of cultures and possibilities available during and after the COVID pandemic.

The contribution by Marissa Willcox, Anna Hickey-Moody and Anne M. Harris builds on the literature on social prescribing to examine therapeutic forms of arts practice and issues of ethics of care on the Instagram Live platform (Chapter 10). The entanglements between performers, audiences, the creation of community, digital media and affective forces are highlighted in their chapter. In so doing, these authors prompt a discussion around how liveness, sociality and connectivity in musical performances should be understood, arts accessibility as a measure of public health and wellbeing as well as how artists can be better supported throughout the COVID crisis.

The chapters in Part IV ('Healthcare Practices and Systems') move beyond the home setting to focus on how medical practitioners and hospitals dealt with the early months of the COVID crisis. In Chapter 11, Jo Murphy-Lawless explains how COVID disrupted Irish cultural norms. She observes that, for the Irish, among the profoundly stressful consequences of COVID-19 was how they were forced to do death differently. Murphy-Lawless shows how the crisis has made painfully visible the social and economic contradictions of contemporary Ireland, including the effects of years of austerity cuts on the Irish National Health Service.

In Chapter 12, Romain Lutaud, Jeremy K. Ward, Gaëtan Gentile and Pierre Verger focus on general practitioners in France and the controversial drug hydroxychloroquine that was initially touted as a preventive agent and treatment for COVID patients. Stepping back to take a longer view, the authors contextualise their case study within the broader politically fraught environment of general practitioners and health authorities in France over more than two decades, which has led to a lack of trust on the part of practitioners in these authorities. They also show how patients' demands on their GPs can lead the practitioners to try new drug therapies such as hydroxychloroquine in situations such as the emergence of this new infectious disease where medical knowledge was still forming.

Anna Sendra, Jordi Farré, Alessandro Lovari and Linda Lombi (Chapter 13) compare the effects of the COVID crisis in Spain and Italy: both countries that were among the hardest hit in the early months of the pandemic. They identify similarities based on what they characterise as a Latin or Mediterranean approach to life, involving close physical proximity to people, cross-generational sharing of residences and regular socialising in public spaces. They also identify how the effects of the 2008 global financial crisis undermined the healthcare systems of both countries. Together, these sociocultural and infrastructural conditions resulted in both countries experiencing similar effects of the pandemic and being forced to endure long-term severe lockdowns to gain control of the spread of the coronavirus.

Chapter 14, by Karen Willis and Natasha Smallwood, turns to the Australian context and responses by frontline healthcare workers to a survey about their experiences of dealing with COVID-19 and the impacts on their mental health and wellbeing. The sheer weight of stress carried by these healthcare workers is revealed in their answers, as they battled with a situation where they were over-worked and concerned about exposing their family members to coronavirus infection. The survey also identifies the effects of 'spillover': the ways that behaviours, attitudes and experiences carry over from one environment (in this case, the hospital and other healthcare settings) to another (the home).

Part V ('Marginalisation and Discrimination') is the final section of the book. The exacerbation of racial and religious discrimination in various regions is pointed out by several contributors. In Chapter 15, Alex Schenkels, Sakina Loukili and Paul Mutsaers discuss implications for parenting resulting from Dutch government's interventions during COVID, with a focus on the experiences of Muslim families living in the Netherlands. The authors bring together a discussion of how norms of intensive parenting were manifested during COVID lockdown, as parents grappled with how to manage learning from home expectations for their children, with an examination of the ways that Muslim beliefs and organisations framed parenting roles. Muslim parents were faced with juggling anti-Muslim racism and mainstream Dutch parenting expectations together with faith-based pronouncements on how they should parent.

Aggie Yellow Horse (Chapter 16) then discusses what she describes as 'the parallel pandemics of COVID-19 and racism' in the context of the USA. She examines how anti-Asian racism and xenophobia rhetoric as well as reports of hate incidents against Asian Americans began to intensify in the USA early in the COVID outbreak. Yellow Horse argues that understanding how such a rapid increase in racist and xenophobic incidences may affect Asian Americans' physical, mental and social health is important, as racism and xenophobia are fundamental causes of health inequalities in the USA in general and for Asian Americans in particular.

Turning to the problem of ageism, Peta Cook, Cassie Curryer, Susan Banks, Barbara Barbosa Neves, Maho Omori, Annetta Mallon and Jack Lam (Chapter 17) draw on Australian news reporting related to risk and COVID to show how the crisis has laid bare societal discourses based on age differences and stereotypes. In these news reports, young people were frequently framed as healthy, active agents engaging in risky behaviours that endanger their health and that of others. In contrast, older people were typically cast as passive and at risk: and in some extreme cases, as worthless.

Together, these contributions offer a rich account of COVID society. They provide snapshots of what life was like for people in a variety of situations and locations living through the first months of the novel coronavirus crisis, including discussion not only of health-related experiences but also the impact on family, work and social life, and leisure activities. The sociomaterial dimensions of quotidian practices are highlighted: death rituals, dating apps, online musical performances, fitness and exercise practices, the role of windows, healthcare work, parenting children learning at home, moving in public space as a blind person and many more diverse topics are explored. In doing so, the authors surface the feelings of strangeness and challenges to norms of practice that were part of many people's experiences, highlighting the profound affective responses that accompanied the disruption to usual cultural forms of sociality and ritual in the wake of the COVID outbreak and restrictions on movement. The authors show how social relationships and social institutions were suspended, re-invented or transformed while social differences were brought to the fore. At the macro level, the book includes localised and comparative analyses of political, health system and policy responses to the pandemic and highlights the differences in representations and experiences of very different social groups, including people with disabilities, LGBTQI people, Dutch Muslim parents, healthcare workers in France and Australia, young adults living in northern Italy, performing artists and their audiences, exercisers in Australia and New Zealand, the Latin cultures of Spain and Italy, Asian Americans and older people in Australia.

Above all, these chapters bring into focus the importance of acknowledging not only the social, political and cultural contexts of COVID experiences, but also their affective, temporal, geographical and spatial dimensions. Beck's writings on risk society were frequently criticised for their generalisations and assumptions, their lack of cultural specificity and attention to the details of what is was like to live with and make sense of risk (Tulloch and Lupton, 2003). In the first phase of the COVID crisis as it has unfolded, we have already learnt that conditions can change very quickly and that complacency or the urge to adopt quick fixes rather than long-term solutions to contain the spread of the coronavirus simply result in further outbreaks and greater uncertainty about the future. As we move into the next stages of the crisis, maintaining a highly focused approach that acknowledges the complexities, affects and situated nature of lived experiences in COVID society remains a crucial research direction for social researchers.

References

Afsahi A, Beausoleil E, Dean R, et al. (2020) Democracy in a global emergency: five lessons from the COVID-19 pandemic. *Democratic Theory* 7 (2): v–xix.

Al-Ali N (2020) Covid-19 and feminism in the Global South: challenges, initiatives and dilemmas. *European Journal of Women's Studies* 27 (4): 333–347.

Bahn K, Cohen J and van der Meulen Rodgers Y (2020) A feminist perspective on COVID-19 and the value of care work globally. *Gender, Work & Organization* 27 (5): 695–699.

Baker SA, Wade M and Walsh MJ (2020) The challenges of responding to misinformation during a pandemic: content moderation and the limitations of the concept of harm. *Media International Australia* 177 (1): 103–107.

Beck U (1992) *Risk Society: Towards a New Modernity*. London: Sage.

Bhatia M (2020) COVID-19 and BAME Group in the United Kingdom. *The International Journal of Community and Social Development* 2 (2): 269–272.

Bjørkdahl K and Carlsen B (2019) Introduction: pandemics, publics, and politics – staging responses to public health crises. In: Bjørkdahl K and Carlsen B (eds) *Pandemics, Publics, and Politics: Staging Responses to Public Health Crises*. Singapore: Springer, pp. 1–9.

Braidotti R (2020) 'We' are in this together, but we are not one and the same. *Journal of Bioethical Inquiry* 17, 465–469.

Brown P (2020) Studying COVID-19 in light of critical approaches to risk and uncertainty: research pathways, conceptual tools, and some magic from Mary Douglas. *Health, Risk & Society* 22 (1): 1–14.

Chan C and Montt Strabucchi M (2020) Many-faced orientalism: racism and xenophobia in a time of the novel coronavirus in Chile. *Asian Ethnicity*. Epub ahead of print.

Craig L (2020) Coronavirus, domestic labour and care: gendered roles locked down. *Journal of Sociology* 56 (4): 684–692.

Dahiya A (2020) The phenomenology of contagion. *Journal of Bioethical Inquiry* 17: 519–523.

Dalglish SL (2020) COVID-19 gives the lie to global health expertise. *The Lancet* 395 (10231): 1189.

de Kloet J, Lin J and Chow YF (2020) 'We are doing better': biopolitical nationalism and the COVID-19 virus in East Asia. *European Journal of Cultural Studies* 23 (4): 635–640.

Dingwall R, Hoffman LM and Staniland K (2013) Introduction: why a sociology of pandemics? *Sociology of Health & Illness* 35 (2): 167–173.

Du L and Cortez LF (2020) Pandemic tops 10 million cases, 500,000 deaths as momentum grows. Retrieved from www.bloomberg.com/news/articles/2020-06-28/global-covid-19-cases-hit-10-million-as-pandemic-gains-momentum (accessed 14 October 2020).

Egede LE and Walker RJ (2020) Structural racism, social risk factors, and Covid-19 – a dangerous convergence for Black Americans. *New England Journal of Medicine* 383: e77. Retrieved from https://www.nejm.org/doi/full/10.1056/NEJMp2023616 (accessed 7 January 2021).

Everts J (2020) The dashboard pandemic. *Dialogues in Human Geography* 10 (2): 260–264.

Goggin G and Ellis K (2020) Disability, communication, and life itself in the COVID-19 pandemic. *Health Sociology Review* 29 (2): 168–176.

Gugushvili A, Koltai J, Stuckler D, et al. (2020) Votes, populism, and pandemics. *International Journal of Public Health* 65 (6): 721–722.

Haokip T (2020) From 'Chinky' to 'coronavirus': racism against Northeast Indians during the Covid-19 pandemic. *Asian Ethnicity*. Epub ahead of print.

Kitchin R (2020) Civil liberties or public health, or civil liberties and public health? Using surveillance technologies to tackle the spread of COVID-19. *Space and Polity*. Epub ahead of print.

Lupton D (2013) *Risk*. London: Routledge.

Lupton D (2020a) Social research for a COVID and post-COVID world: an initial agenda. Retrieved from https://medium.com/@deborahalupton/social-research-for-a-covid-and-post-covid-world-an-initial-agenda-796868f1fb0e (accessed 14 October 2020).

Lupton D (2020b) Special section on 'Sociology and the Coronavirus (COVID-19) Pandemic'. *Health Sociology Review* 29 (2): 111–112.

Mahase E (2020) Covid-19: What do we know about 'long covid'? *BMJ*, 370. Retrieved from www.bmj.com/content/370/bmj.m2815.abstract (accessed 14 October 2020).

Malta M, Murray L, da Silva CMFP, et al. (2020) Coronavirus in Brazil: the heavy weight of inequality and unsound leadership. *EClinicalMedicine* 25. Retrieved from https://www.thelancet.com/journals/eclinm/article/PIIS2589-5370(20)30216-9/fulltext (accessed 7 January 2021).

Markham F and Smith D (2020) *Indigenous Australians and the COVID 19 Crisis: Perspectives on Public Policy*. Canberra: Australian National University.

Matache M and Bhabha J (2020) Anti-Roma racism is spiraling during COVID-19 pandemic. *Health and Human Rights* 22 (1): 379–382.

Meese J, Frith J and Wilken R (2020) COVID-19, 5G conspiracies and infrastructural futures. *Media International Australia* 177 (1): 30–46.

Meijer A, Webster CWR, et al. (2020) The COVID-19-crisis and the information polity: An overview of responses and discussions in twenty-one countries from six continents. *Information Polity* 25 (3): 243–274.

Milan S and Treré E (2020) The rise of the data poor: the COVID-19 pandemic seen from the margins. *Social Media + Society* 6. Retrieved from https://journals.sagepub.com/doi/full/10.1177/2056305120948233 (accessed 7 January 2021).

Nguyen MH, Gruber J, Fuchs J, et al. (2020) Changes in digital communication during the COVID-19 global pandemic: implications for digital inequality and future research. *Social Media + Society*, 6. Retrieved from https://journals.sagepub.com/doi/full/10.1177/2056305120948255 (accessed 7 January 2021).

Orso D, Federici N, Copetti R, et al. (2020) Infodemic and the spread of fake news in the COVID-19 era. *European Journal of Emergency Medicine* 27: 327–328.

Pang B (2020) Beyond hypervisibility and fear: British Chinese communities' leisure and health-related experiences in the time of coronavirus. *Leisure Sciences*. Epub ahead of print.

Pierre J (2020) Nudges against pandemics: Sweden's COVID-19 containment strategy in perspective. *Policy and Society* 39 (3): 478–493.

Pleyers G (2020) A plea for global sociology in times of the coronavirus. Retrieved from www.isa-sociology.org/frontend/web/uploads/files/Global%20Sociology%20in%20Times%20of%20the%20Coronavirus.pdf (accessed 14 October 2020).

Rahman SY (2020) 'Social distancing' during COVID-19: the metaphors and politics of pandemic response in India. *Health Sociology Review* 29 (2): 131–139.

Rambaree K and Nässén N (2020) 'The Swedish Strategy' to COVID-19 pandemic: impact on vulnerable and marginalised communities. *The International Journal of Community and Social Development* 2 (2): 234–250.

Roberto KJ, Johnson AF and Rauhaus BM (2020) Stigmatization and prejudice during the COVID-19 pandemic. *Administrative Theory & Praxis* 42 (3): 364–378.

Rocco P, Béland D and Waddan A (2020) Stuck in neutral? Federalism, policy instruments, and counter-cyclical responses to COVID-19 in the United States. *Policy and Society* 39 (3): 458–477.

Rodrigues UM and Xu J (2020) Regulation of COVID-19 fake news infodemic in China and India. *Media International Australia* 177 (1): 125–131.

Scambler G (2020) Covid-19 as a 'breaching experiment': exposing the fractured society. *Health Sociology Review* 29 (2): 140–148.

Searle A and Turnbull J (2020) Resurgent natures? More-than-human perspectives on COVID-19. *Dialogues in Human Geography* 10 (2): 291–295.

Shimizu K (2020) 2019-nCoV, fake news, and racism. *The Lancet* 395 (10225): 685–686.

Strong P (1990) Epidemic psychology: a model. *Sociology of Health & Illness* 12 (3): 249–259.

Thomson K (2020) By the light of the corona (virus): revealing hegemonic masculinity and the double bind for men in responding to crises. *Health Sociology Review* 29 (2): 149–157.

Tulloch J and Lupton D (2003) *Risk and Everyday Life*. London: Sage.

van Loon J (2005) Epidemic space. *Critical Public Health* 15 (1): 39–52.

Watson A, Lupton D and Michael M (2020) Enacting intimacy and sociality at a distance in the COVID-19 crisis: the sociomaterialities of home-based communication technologies. *Media International Australia*. Epub ahead of print.

Williamson E, Lombard N and Brooks-Hay O (2020) Domestic violence and abuse, coronavirus, and the media narrative. *Journal of Gender-Based Violence* 4 (2): 289–294.

World Health Organization (2020) WHO timeline – COVID-19. Retrieved from www.who.int/news-room/detail/27-04-2020-who-timeline—covid-19 (accessed 14 October 2020).

2

CONTEXTUALISING COVID-19

Sociocultural perspectives on contagion

Deborah Lupton

Introduction

When serious infection disease outbreaks occur, many routine dimensions of everyday life can be thrown into disarray, as uncertainty, fear and anxiety are heightened, rapid changes are made and restrictions are imposed in the attempt to thwart the spread of contagion. In understanding and dealing with the COVID-19 crisis, we have much to learn from the previous literature concerning how societies have responded to previous epidemics and pandemics. Sociologists, social historians and other social researchers have been devoting attention to the sociocultural dimensions of contagion for some time, identifying the broader contexts in which outbreaks of infectious disease take place. From this perspective, contagion is always a social phenomenon, infused with and understood through situated and shifting meanings and practices. Writing at the peak of the HIV/AIDS crisis, medical historian Charles Rosenberg (1988: 327) observed that epidemics serve as 'mirrors held up to society in which more general patterns of social values and attitudes appear in sharp relief'. Similarly, responding to the question they set themselves for a special issue on the topic – 'Why a sociology of pandemics?' – Dingwall et al. (2013) note that when health crises such as pandemics are emerging, aspects of societies that might otherwise be taken for granted or hidden, such as entrenched social inequalities and social marginalisation, often come starkly to the fore.

This chapter provides such an overview, establishing the basis for the remainder of this book on the social aspects of the COVID pandemic by 'setting the scene'. I begin by describing how the COVID pandemic is the latest of a long line of new and re-emerging infectious disease outbreaks occurring since the 1970s. I then introduce the major approaches that have been used to interpret and explain the sociocultural effects of and responses to these outbreaks and earlier epidemics and pandemics. Across this literature, social histories, political economy perspectives, social constructionism and risk theory, along with Foucauldian theory have predominated. More recently, postcolonial and sociomaterial analyses have appeared. I provide examples of how these approaches have been taken up in the literature and summarise the major themes that have emerged.

New and re-emerging infectious diseases

Severe outbreaks of infectious diseases such as influenza, cholera, plague, typhus, smallpox and yellow fever once played a major role in causing serious illness and early death in human populations (Mack, 1991; Bashford, 2016). Their impact has gradually diminished over the past century (particularly in middle-income and high-income countries) with the introduction of better sanitation and hygienic measures, the generation and application of scientific knowledge of how infection is caused and spread, and the invention and application of pharmaceuticals and widespread vaccination programmes (Arrizabalaga, 2016; Rosenberg, 1988). The success of these measures inspired the World Health Organization (WHO) to optimistically announce in its 'Global Strategy for Health for All by the Year 2000' (World Health Organization 1981) that it aimed to prevent the spread of the most infectious diseases by the end of the 20th century through universal healthcare and vaccination programmes.

Since the late 20th century, however, new or re-emerging infectious diseases have begun to have a significant impact on human health and mortality rates once more (Arrizabalaga, 2016; McCloskey et al., 2014). Cases of the deadly Ebola virus were first recorded in the Democratic Republic of Congo in 1976, the same year that a legionella (Legionnaires' disease) outbreak, involving a pneumonia-type condition, was recorded in the USA (Arrizabalaga, 2016). HIV/AIDS, the initial cases of which were reported in the US in 1981, was the first of these new diseases to receive world attention. WHO characterises HIV/AIDS as 'a major global public health issue' (World Health Organization, 2020a). WHO's website documents that by the end of 2018, an estimated 38 million people worldwide were living with HIV/AIDS, with an accumulated total of 33 million deaths from the condition.

Outbreaks of various new or re-emerging infectious diseases occurring from the end of the 20th century, such as West Nile virus (sporadic outbreaks from 1999 onwards), severe acute respiratory syndrome (SARS) (2003), avian influenza (2003–2007), swine influenza (H1N1) (2009), Middle East respiratory syndrome (MERS) (2012 onwards), Ebola virus disease (2014–2016) and Zika virus disease (2015–2016), have instigated concern about how viral contagion has occurred between humans and the role played by other animals in these infection networks. Observing and responding to these previous outbreaks, several commentators and organisations had begun to warn of the inevitability that an even more serious new pandemic was waiting in the wings, and that all nations should be preparing for it (Ball, 2020; Garrett, 1994). A slew of popular films such as *Outbreak* and *Contagion* have depicted exactly this scenario and its grave consequences for humanity (Lynteris, 2016).

Medical and public health experts and organisations have long called for an ecological perspective on emerging diseases, often referred to as the One Health or planetary health approach, in which human health is viewed as inextricably interrelated with another animals' health and that of other living creatures in the global ecosystem (McCloskey et al., 2014; Horton et al., 2014; Rock and Degeling, 2015; Chien, 2013). By 1994, WHO had created a programme on emerging infectious diseases, emphasising that globalisation had created the conditions for the rapid dispersal of such diseases around the world (Arrizabalaga, 2016). In 2015, a panel of scientists and public health experts convened by WHO met in Geneva to create a priority list of 'the top five to ten emerging pathogens likely to cause severe outbreaks in the near future, and for which few or no medical countermeasures exist'. The disease priorities listed as needing urgent research and development attention were Crimean Congo haemorrhagic fever, Ebola, Marburg virus disease, Lassa fever, MERS and SARS, Nipah virus disease and Rift Valley fever (World Health Organization, 2015).

COVID, caused by a novel coronavirus (SARS CoV-2), is the latest – and to date, most momentous – emerging infectious disease. At first presenting at the end of 2019 as an atypical pneumonia-like condition among a small number of cases in the Chinese city of Wuhan (World Health Organization, 2020c), it has since become apparent that COVID can dangerously affect other systems and organs, and that survivors often experience ill-effects of the disease for months (or possibly long term) (Argenziano et al., 2020). The coronavirus has spread rapidly around the world. WHO announced that COVID was declared a pandemic on 11 March 2020 – just over two months after the first cases were reported. By the end of July 2020, over 14 million cases of COVID had been reported worldwide, with over half a million deaths. At that point in the pandemic, the US, Brazil and India had become the most affected countries, accounting for more than a quarter of all confirmed cases globally (Tanne, 2020).

While the COVID pandemic shares some similarities with previous pandemics in terms of sociocultural and political responses, there are a number of significant differences. Unlike HIV/AIDS, the coronavirus is not associated with stigmatised social practices such as sexual behaviour or injecting drug use. Rather, it is spread far more universally (and dangerously) in the air as aerosol viral particles from coughing, sneezing or even speaking and breathing and by touching objects on which such particles may settle (World Health Organization, 2020b). While previous influenza pandemics of the past two decades have involved similar modes of transmission, they were far less contagious than the coronavirus, and were much more easily contained geographically, to the point that some critics claimed that warnings concerning their potential health and economic effects were overblown and alarmist (Bjørkdahl and Carlsen, 2019).

In contrast, it is hard to overstate the extent to which the COVID outbreak has affected the world. All social groups, across all geographical regions, are at risk from contracting the coronavirus if they leave their homes and mingle with potentially infected known or unknown people. Unlike any of the more recent pandemics,

COVID control requires people who are not designated as 'essential workers' to spend long periods of isolation in their homes to protect against infection, which, in turn, has caused massive economic downturns. More than a health problem, COVID is a global crisis on a large scale. It has seriously affected all world regions, wreaking devastation on national economies and disrupting social life. Some of the wealthiest and most powerful nations have been among the most badly affected: the US reported the greatest number of infections and death rates in the first six months (Tanne, 2020).

The scale of COVID, therefore, eclipses any of the pandemics emerging over the past 50 years, and can best be compared with the Spanish influenza pandemic that took place a century ago, infecting one-third of the world's population and killing an estimated 50–100 million people (Flecknoe et al., 2018). Even then, there are many differences, given the intensification of processes of globalisation that have occurred over that century, such as the mass movements of people across the globe through the expansion of air travel, resulting in the coronavirus spreading much more quickly than did Spanish influenza. The groups at risk from Spanish influenza were also very different: there were many young people among the afflicted and dead, whereas, thus far, the coronavirus has overwhelmingly had its worst effects on older people (Aassve et al., 2020).

Sociocultural analyses of pandemics

Social histories of responses to infectious disease outbreaks have drawn attention to the continuing discrimination and stigmatisation of social groups who have been identified as 'contaminating' and posing a risk to others, often involving moral judgements about their worth and value as humans (Nelkin and Gilman, 1991; Rosenberg, 1988). *Political economy approaches*, building on Marxist theory, highlight the macro-political dimensions of health risks in contemporary societies. They seek to identify socioeconomic structures and inequalities affecting health status across social groups, focusing on the relationship between health and gender, age, social class, education level and race/ethnicity (Doyal and Pennell, 1979; Raphael, 2013). *Social constructionism* views health and illness as embodied states that are defined, understood and managed through worldviews, beliefs and meanings that are always historically and culturally situated. From this perspective, viruses are conceptualised as assemblages of biological matter, discourses and power relations (Conrad and Barker, 2010; Bury, 1986).

Scholars engaging with *Foucauldian theory*, and particularly his concepts of governmentality, biopower and biopolitics, seek to surface the complex relations of power that are inherent in social responses to disease. These power relations produce knowledges, discourses, practices and norms about human bodies and operate to manage populations, including encouraging people to engage in self-care and self-discipline to manage health and illness as part of being ideal citizens (Lupton, 1995; Keshet and Popper-Giveon, 2018). *Risk theory* also incorporates Foucauldian perspectives, but the scholarship of Ulrich Beck and Mary Douglas is also highly influential (Lupton, 2013). Beck's risk society thesis (Beck 1992), and particularly his concept of 'world risk society' (Beck 1999), focuses on the ways in which risk is dispersed across international borders as part of the processes of modernisation, individualisation and globalisation. Douglas's (1992; Douglas and Wildavsky, 1982) work on risk takes an anthropological perspective, focusing on the cultural aspects and the ways that concepts of Self and Other are reproduced and maintained during times of health crises to enforce symbolic boundaries that help people feel safe.

Drawing on theorists such as Gayatri Spivak, Edward Said and Homi Bhabha (Bhambra, 2014), *postcolonial perspectives* on health and medicine devote attention to the persistent racism and Othering that is evident in the legacy of colonial histories and the continuing fraught relationships between settler groups and Indigenous and First Nations peoples (King, 2002). The *sociomaterial perspective* draws on science and technology studies, affect theory, new materialism and cultural geographies (Andrews and Duff, 2019). These analyses have sought to identify the more-than-human health and illness assemblages that emerge when people, other living things and non-living things come together, and the vitalities and forces that are generated with and through these assemblages (Lupton, 2019).

The emergence of the HIV/AIDS in the early 1980s stimulated a plethora of social and cultural analyses concerning the representation of risk and the stigmatisation and marginalisation of social groups such as gay men, injecting drug users and sex workers. Given that HIV is spread through very close physical contact and the exchange of body fluids such as blood and semen during activities such as penetrative sex and the sharing of needles to inject drugs, it was constantly associated with connotations of deviance, victim-blaming and moral judgements. Regardless of how they contracted HIV, people living with the virus were frequently ostracised and subjected to stigma, particularly if it was assumed that they had engaged in 'deviant' behaviours (Lupton, 1994, 1999; Brandt, 1991; Brown, 2000; Carter and Watney, 1989; Crawford, 1994; Patton, 1986). As the epidemic began to spread from the US and other high-income countries to other regions of the world, HIV/AIDS was also one of the first infectious disease outbreaks to attract the application of theories of globalisation, modernity and risk (Bancroft, 2001; Douglas and Calvez, 1990).

Many subsequent social analyses of epidemics and pandemics have identified the ways that risk has been associated with the othering of marginalised social groups: often involving moral judgements about lack of personal responsibility. A study of SARS-related stigma among a group of Hong Kong residents living in the heart of an outbreak (Lee et al., 2005) found that participants reported high levels of distress from being shunned, insulted, marginalised and rejected by others in their city. Gendered concepts of responsibility for protecting others against risk were identified in a sociohistorical study of the Canadian experience of the Spanish flu pandemic. The researchers found that women were portrayed as having a duty of care for people who have become ill from infectious diseases, thus being placed in the front-line of healthcare and at greater risk of infection themselves (Godderis and Rossiter, 2013). Racism is frequently part of social responses to disease outbreaks.

The othering of Africans in the American media's portrayal of the Ebola epidemic (Monson, 2017) and social media positioning of national governments and public health authorities as well as Africans as figures of blame during this epidemic (Roy et al., 2020) have been noted in the social research literature. In contrast, epidemiologists have emerged as unlikely heroes in popular cultural portrayals such as films depicting fictional disease outbreaks (Lynteris, 2016).

Numerous analyses of news and social media coverage of outbreaks of avian influenza (Abeysinghe and White, 2011), swine influenza (Staniland and Smith, 2013; Mesch et al., 2013), SARS (Lewison, 2008), Zika (Ribeiro et al., 2018; Fabrício, 2019) and Ebola (Kilgo et al., 2019; Roy et al., 2020) have also demonstrated the social construction of risk and notions of responsibility. For example, an investigation into the Brazilian news media's coverage of the Zika outbreaks (Ribeiro et al., 2018) found that the 'war' metaphor was used to frame the social representations and policy responses. The gendered and other socio-economic impacts of the Zika outbreak in Brazil were largely overlooked in that country's news reporting. The focus was on the importance of eradicating the vector of the virus (mosquitoes) and the expectation that pregnant women would take responsibility to avoid infection to protect their foetuses.

Macro-political critiques have involved a range of theoretical perspectives. A sociological analysis of avian influenza control in Vietnam engaged with Beck's risk society approach, arguing that the globalisation of risk as evidenced by such outbreaks has pushed nations to adopt a more cosmopolitan approach to health policy (Figuié, 2013). A critical analysis of the Ebola virus outbreaks in West Africa is an example of the political economy approach used together with postcolonial theory (Obeng-Odoom and Bockarie, 2018). A discussion of the response to the 2004 West Nile virus outbreak by Canadian authorities, (Gislason, 2013) adopted a social constructionist and Foucauldian analysis to identify the various techniques and technologies of power that were demonstrated: surveillance, normalisation, exclusion and regulation.

While nowhere near comparable to the outpouring of sociocultural research on HIV/AIDS, the 2009 swine flu pandemic attracted some degree of attention from social researchers. This pandemic provides an interesting comparison with the current COVID crisis. What is notable about the swine flu outbreak is that at first it threatened to become serious, but in the end proved to be much milder than expected (Davis et al., 2014). Sociologists examined such topics as how Australian publics' behaviour and their vulnerability to the pandemic was expressed in health policy (Stephenson et al., 2014; Davis et al., 2011), British public health authorities' anticipatory actions (Barker, 2012) and their reflections on how well they handled the situation (Davis et al., 2014). Other issues examined included the over-reliance on speculative modelling during the swine flu pandemic (Chambers et al., 2012), publics' attitudes to vaccination (Carlsen and Glenton, 2016) and the role of blame and inequities in risk management and access to medicines globally during that pandemic (Sparke and Anguelov, 2012). More broadly, Australian and British publics' concepts of personal risk (Davis et al., 2015; Lohm et al., 2015) and immunity (Davis et al., 2015; Davis, 2019) in the face of recent influenza epidemics and pandemics have also been canvassed.

Given that many of the latest pandemics, including COVID, are zoonotic (spread by an animal host to humans), sociomaterialist perspectives offer important insights into the complex entanglements of human health and wellbeing with other animals and other living things. A sociomaterialist perspective on planetary health devotes attention to the logics, knowledge practices and sociocultural and socio-spatial dimensions, including issues of neoliberalist politics, postcolonialism, racism, gender and other forms of othering that are often left unacknowledged by medical and public health visions of One Health (Hinchliffe, 2015). The space and place in which contagious agents such as viruses and bacteria assemble with humans and other animals are also identified as key elements of viral assemblages (Hinchliffe, 2015). Ethnographic work that focuses on the lived experiences of people working with animals in environments where epidemics and pandemics emerge has pointed to the micro-political dimensions of the entanglements of humans with nonhumans. For example, an ethnography of responses to avian influenza in Vietnam (Porter, 2013) brought together the Foucauldian concept of biopower with a multispecies approach to extend the concept of One Health. As this ethnography demonstrated, in the case of avian influenza, the living arrangements of people with poultry were central to the conduits of contagion. Identifying these multispecies relations can work towards breaking the contagious circuit.

The concept of 'epidemic space' (van Loon, 2005) also draws attention to the spatial and other material dimensions of more-than-human relations and assemblages. Social histories of medicine have demonstrated how material things and space and place have been central to responses to infectious disease outbreaks, involving the identification and disciplining of 'at risk' or 'risky groups. Exclusionary and isolation practices are frequently the mode by which such 'problem populations' have been disciplined and contained (Bashford and Strange, 2003). Quarantine is one such measure, undertaken since the 14th century to deal with outbreaks of the plague and proliferating over the 19th and 20th centuries (Bashford, 2016). Practices of disinfection, infectious disease surveillance and contact tracing emerged in the 19th century, with citizens encouraged to take responsibility for hygienic practices in both public and domestic spaces (Mooney, 2015). The use of face masks to prevent against infection has been traced back to the 1910–11 Manchurian plague outbreak, following new scientific knowledge that the plague virus could be airborne (Lynteris, 2018).

Concluding comments

This brief overview of previous sociocultural research into epidemics and pandemics has identified major themes in social, cultural and historical responses to contagion. Sociocultural research has highlighted the ways that broad social changes such as globalisation and modernisation have created the conditions for the emergence of the COVID crisis. The role played by social group membership and socioeconomic status in configuring people's experiences of pandemics and their exposure to infection has been identified. The literature has provided valuable insights into the ways that risk and risk groups have been portrayed in policy documents, news, social media and other popular media, how certain voices have received attention while others have been excluded, blamed or marginalised and how dominant metaphors and social imaginaries have been reproduced. Further, this body of work has surfaced the micro-political aspects of more-than-human assemblages of contagion and embodiment, including affective, temporal, material, spatial and multispecies dimensions. Analyses of the COVID crisis should acknowledge and build on this research, taking inspiration from the valuable insights that are offered and working to contextualise the current pandemic within its frameworks.

References

Aassve A, Alfani G, Gandolfi F and Le Moglie M (2020) Pandemics and social capital: from the Spanish flu of 1918–19 to COVID-19. Retrieved from https://voxeu.org/article/pandemics-and-social-capital (accessed 8 August 2020).

Abeysinghe S and White K (2011) The avian influenza pandemic: discourses of risk, contagion and preparation in Australia. *Health, Risk & Society* 13 (4): 311–326.

Andrews GJ and Duff C (2019) Matter beginning to matter: on posthumanist understandings of the vital emergence of health. *Social Science & Medicine* 226: 123–134.

Argenziano MG, Bruce SL, Slater CL et al. (2020) Characterization and clinical course of 1000 patients with coronavirus disease 2019 in New York: retrospective case series. *British Medical Journal* 369. Retrieved from www.bmj.com/content/369/bmj.m1996.abstract (accessed 15 August 2020).

Arrizabalaga J (2016) The global threat of (re)emerging diseases: contesting the adequacy of biomedical discourse and practice. In: Davis JE and Gonzalez AM (eds) *To Fix or to Heal: Patient Care, Public Health, and the Limits of Biomedicine*. New York: New York University Press, pp. 177–207.

Ball P (2020) Pandemic science and politics. *The Lancet* 396 (10246): 229–230.

Bancroft A (2001) Globalisation and HIV/AIDS: inequality and the boundaries of a symbolic epidemic. *Health, Risk & Society* 3 (1): 89–98.

Barker K (2012) Influenza preparedness and the bureaucratic reflex: anticipating and generating the 2009 H1N1 event. *Health & Place* 18 (4): 701–709.

Bashford A (2016) *Quarantine: Local and Global Histories*. London: Palgrave.

Bashford A and Strange C (2003) Isolation and exclusion in the modern world. In: Bashford A and Strange C (eds) *Isolation: Places and Practices of Exclusion*. London: Routledge, pp.1–21.

Beck U (1992) *Risk Society: Towards a New Modernity*. London: Sage.

Beck U (1999) *World Risk Society*. Malden, MA: Polity Press.

Bhambra GK (2014) Postcolonial and decolonial dialogues. *Postcolonial Studies* 17 (2): 115–121.

Bjørkdahl K and Carlsen B (2019) Introduction: pandemics, publics, and politics – staging responses to public health crises. In: Bjørkdahl K and Carlsen B (eds) *Pandemics, Publics, and Politics: Staging Responses to Public Health Crises*. Singapore: Springer, pp. 1–9.

Brandt A (1991) AIDS and metaphor: toward the social meaning of epidemic disease. In: Mack A (ed) *In Time of Plague: The History and Social Consequences of Lethal Epidemic Disease*. New York: New York University Press, pp. 91–110.

Brown T (2000) AIDS, risk and social governance. *Social Science & Medicine* 50 (9): 1273–1284.

Bury MR (1986) Social constructionism and the development of medical sociology. *Sociology of Health & Illness* 8 (2): 137–169.

Carlsen B and Glenton C (2016) The swine flu vaccine, public attitudes, and researcher interpretations: a systematic review of qualitative research. *BMC Health Services Research* 16. Retrieved from https://bmchealthservres.biomedcentral.com/articles/10.1186/s12913-016-1466-7 (accessed 7 January 2021).

Carter E and Watney S (1989) *Taking Liberties: AIDS and Cultural Politics*. London: Serpent's Tail.

Chambers J, Barker K and Rouse A (2012) Reflections on the UK's approach to the 2009 swine flu pandemic: conflicts between national government and the local management of the public health response. *Health & Place* 18 (4): 737–745.

Chien Y-J (2013) How did international agencies perceive the avian influenza problem? The adoption and manufacture of the 'One World, One Health' framework. *Sociology of Health & Illness* 35 (2): 213–226.

Conrad P and Barker KK (2010) The social construction of illness: key insights and policy implications. *Journal of Health and Social Behavior* 51 (1_suppl): S67–S79.

Crawford R (1994) The boundaries of the self and the unhealthy other: reflections on health, culture and AIDS. *Social Science & Medicine* 38 (10): 1347–1365.

Davis M (2019) Uncertainty and immunity in public communications on pandemics. In: Bjørkdahl K and Carlsen B (eds) *Pandemics, Publics, and Politics: Staging Responses to Public Health Crises*. Singapore: Springer, pp. 29–42.

Davis M, Flowers P, Lohm D, Waller E and Stephenson N (2015) Immunity, biopolitics and pandemics: public and individual responses to the threat to life. *Body & Society* 22 (4): 130–154.

Davis M, Flowers P and Stephenson N (2014) 'We had to do what we thought was right at the time': retrospective discourse on the 2009 H1N1 pandemic in the UK. *Sociology of Health & Illness* 36 (3): 369–382.

Davis M, Stephenson N and Flowers P (2011) Compliant, complacent or panicked? Investigating the problematisation of the Australian general public in pandemic influenza control. *Social Science & Medicine* 72 (6): 912–918.

Dingwall R, Hoffman LM and Staniland K (2013) Introduction: why a sociology of pandemics? *Sociology of Health & Illness* 35 (2): 167–173.

Douglas M (1992) *Risk and Blame: Essays in Cultural Theory*. London: Routledge.

Douglas M and Calvez M (1990) The self as risk taker: a cultural theory of contagion in relation to AIDS. *The Sociological Review* 38 (3): 445–464.

Douglas M and Wildavsky A (1982) *Risk and Culture: An Essay on the Selection of Technological and Environmental Dangers*. Berkeley, CA: University of California Press.

Doyal L and Pennell I (1979) *The Political Economy of Health*. London: Pluto Press.

Fabrício BF (2019) Discourse circulation in news coverage of the Zika virus outbreak: colonial geopolitics, biomediatization and affect. *Discourse, Context & Media* 30. Retrieved from https://doi.org/10.1016/j.dcm.2019.01.002 (accessed 7 January 2021).

Figuié M (2013) Global health risks and cosmopolitisation: from emergence to interference. *Sociology of Health & Illness* 35 (2): 227–240.

Flecknoe D, Charles Wakefield B and Simmons A (2018) Plagues & wars: the 'Spanish Flu' pandemic as a lesson from history. *Medicine, Conflict and Survival* 34 (2): 61–68.

Garrett L (1994) *The Coming Plague: Newly Emerging Diseases in a World Out of Balance*. London: Penguin.

Gislason MK (2013) West Nile virus: the production of a public health pandemic. *Sociology of Health & Illness* 35 (2): 188–199.

Godderis R and Rossiter K (2013) 'If you have a soul, you will volunteer at once': gendered expectations of duty to care during pandemics. *Sociology of Health & Illness* 35 (2): 304–308.

Hinchliffe S (2015) More than one world, more than one health: re-configuring interspecies health. *Social Science & Medicine* 129: 28–35.

Horton R, Beaglehole R, Bonita R, Raeburn J, McKee M and Wall S (2014) From public to planetary health: a manifesto. *The Lancet* 383 (9920): 847.

Keshet Y and Popper-Giveon A (2018) The undisciplined patient in neoliberal society: conscious, informed and intuitive health behaviours. *Health, Risk & Society* 20(3–4): 182–199.

Kilgo DK, Yoo J and Johnson TJ (2019) Spreading Ebola panic: newspaper and social media coverage of the 2014 Ebola health crisis. *Health Communication* 34 (8): 811–817.

King NB (2002) Security, disease, commerce: ideologies of postcolonial global health. *Social Studies of Science* 32(5–6): 763–789.

Lee S, Chan LYY, Chau AMY, Kwok KPS and Kleinman A (2005) The experience of SARS-related stigma at Amoy Gardens. *Social Science & Medicine* 61 (9): 2038–2046.

Lewison G (2008) The reporting of the risks from severe acute respiratory syndrome (SARS) in the news media, 2003–2004. *Health, Risk & Society* 10 (3): 241–262.

Lohm D, Davis M, Flowers P and Stephenson N (2015) 'Fuzzy' virus: indeterminate influenza biology, diagnosis and surveillance in the risk ontologies of the general public in time of pandemics. *Health, Risk & Society* 17 (2): 115–131.

Lupton D (1994) *Moral Threats and Dangerous Desires: AIDS in the News Media*. Bristol: Taylor & Francis.

Lupton D (1995) *The Imperative of Health: Public Health and the Regulated Body*. London: Sage.

Lupton D (1999) Archetypes of infection: people with HIV/AIDS in the Australian press in the mid 1990s. *Sociology of Health & Illness* 21 (1): 37–53.

Lupton D (2013) *Risk*. London: Routledge.

Lupton D (2019) Toward a more-than-human analysis of digital health: inspirations from feminist new materialism. *Qualitative Health Research* 29 (14): 1998–2009.

Lynteris C (2016) The epidemiologist as culture hero: visualizing humanity in the age of 'the next pandemic'. *Visual Anthropology* 29 (1): 36–53.

Lynteris C (2018) Plague masks: the visual emergence of anti-epidemic personal protection equipment. *Medical Anthropology* 37 (6): 442–457.

Mack A (1991) *In Time of Plague: The History and Social Consequences of Lethal Epidemic Disease*. New York: NYU Press.

McCloskey B, Dar O, Zumla A and Heymann DL (2014) Emerging infectious diseases and pandemic potential: status quo and reducing risk of global spread. *The Lancet Infectious Diseases* 14 (10): 1001–1010.

Mesch GS, Schwirian KP and Kolobov T (2013) Attention to the media and worry over becoming infected: the case of the Swine Flu (H1N1) Epidemic of 2009. *Sociology of Health & Illness* 35 (2): 325–331.

Monson S (2017) Ebola as African: American media discourses of panic and otherization. *Africa Today* 63 (3): 3–27.

Mooney G (2015) *Intrusive Interventions: Public Health, Domestic Space, and Infectious Disease Surveillance in England, 1840–1914*. Rochester: University of Rochester Press.

Nelkin D and Gilman S (1991) Placing blame for devastating disease. In: Mack A (ed.) *In Time of Plague: The History and Social Consequences of Lethal Epidemic Disease*. New York: New York University Press, pp.39–56.

Obeng-Odoom F and Bockarie MMB (2018) The political economy of the Ebola virus disease. *Social Change* 48 (1): 18–35.

Patton C (1986) *Sex and Germs: The Politics of AIDS*. Montreal: Black Rose Books.

Porter N (2013) Bird flu biopower: Strategies for multispecies coexistence in Việt Nam. *American Ethnologist* 40 (1): 132–148.

Raphael D (2013) The political economy of health promotion: part 1, national commitments to provision of the prerequisites of health. *Health Promotion International* 28 (1): 95–111.

Ribeiro B, Hartley S, Nerlich B and Jaspal R (2018) Media coverage of the Zika crisis in Brazil: the construction of a 'war'frame that masked social and gender inequalities. *Social Science & Medicine* 200: 137–144.

Rock MJ and Degeling C (2015) Public health ethics and more-than-human solidarity. *Social Science & Medicine* 129: 61–67.

Rosenberg CE (1988) The definition and control of disease – an introduction. *Social Research* 55 (3): 327–330.

Roy M, Moreau N, Rousseau C, Mercier A, Wilson A and Atlani-Duault L (2020) Ebola and localized blame on social media: analysis of Twitter and Facebook conversations during the 2014–2015 Ebola epidemic. *Culture, Medicine, and Psychiatry* 44 (1): 56–79.

Sparke M and Anguelov D (2012) H1N1, globalization and the epidemiology of inequality. *Health & Place* 18 (4): 726–736.

Staniland K and Smith G (2013) Flu frames. *Sociology of Health & Illness* 35 (2): 309–324.

Stephenson N, Davis M, Flowers P, MacGregor C and Waller E (2014) Mobilising 'vulnerability' in the public health response to pandemic influenza. *Social Science & Medicine* 102: 10–17.

Tanne JH (2020) Covid-19: US sees record rise in cases. *British Medical Journal* 370. Retrieved from www.bmj.com/content/370/bmj.m2676.abstract (accessed 28 August 2020).

Van Loon J (2005) Epidemic space. *Critical Public Health* 15 (1): 39–52.

World Health Organization (1981) Global strategy for health for all by the year 2000. Available at: https://apps.who.int/iris/bitstream/handle/10665/38893/9241800038.pdf;jsessionid=0466F0DF59D3966A9F639C77A02ACB94?sequence=1 (accessed 20 August 2020).

World Health Organization (2015) WHO publishes list of top emerging diseases likely to cause major epidemics. Retrieved from www.who.int/medicines/ebola-treatment/WHO-list-of-top-emerging-diseases/en/ (accessed 20 August 2020).

World Health Organization (2020a) HIV/AIDS. Retrieved from www.who.int/news-room/fact-sheets/detail/hiv-aids (accessed 20 August 2020).

World Health Organization (2020b) Q&A: how is COVID-19 transmitted? Retrieved from www.who.int/emergencies/diseases/novel-coronavirus-2019/question-and-answers-hub/q-a-detail/q-a-how-is-covid-19-transmitted?gclid=CjwKCAjwsO_4BRBBEiwAyagRTTfHZ6hw7Q_pj5sMNnF8i5biRxj4b3polusXYBPGsmVNim03RwLbNxoC8R8QAvD_BwE (accessed 20 August 2020).

World Health Organization (2020c) WHO timeline – COVID-19. Retrieved from www.who.int/news-room/detail/27-04-2020-who-timeline—covid-19 (accessed 28 August 2020).

PART II

Space, the body and mobilities

3

MOVING TARGET, MOVING PARTS

The multiple mobilities of the COVID-19 pandemic

Nicola Burns, Luca Follis, Karolina Follis and Janine Morley

Introduction

In the COVID-19 pandemic, humans are disease vectors. The coronavirus spreads rapidly, riding the crest of human mobility and movement. It forces a dramatic public health imperative: stop moving, stay at home, keep your distance. In the spring of 2020, most governments in the Global North and in many other regions introduced far-reaching restrictions on human movement. These measures affected mobility at all levels, from the suspension of daily commutes, to the closure of international borders, the grounding of flights, the imposition of quarantine, the halting of humanitarian missions and the suspension of normal asylum procedures. If the story of globalisation thus far has largely been one of accelerating mobilities of capital, objects, information and humans (Urry, 2007), the pandemic altered its course.

The mobilities paradigm, that is the sociological focus on the movement of human and non-human actors, offers a means by which to explore the dynamic geography of this emergency by mapping its scalar projection from the body to the local areas and global sites where the restless movement of ideas, people and things is enacted (Cresswell, 2010). The crisis has been characterised by the interruption, disruption and arrestment of mobility, as well as an attention to the circulation of people and things at society's most granular level (i.e. households), highlighting new inequalities and shining a light on older ones. In this chapter, we draw on the mobilities paradigm to map the UK's COVID response and illustrate how inequalities in mobility, interwoven in different sites and at different scales – micro, meso and macro – generated cascades of systemic failure that limited the effectiveness of local and national responses, evident in the fact that during the first half of 2020 the UK had the highest excess mortality rate in Europe (Office for National Statistics, 2020).

We begin our essay by looking at the micro scale of local impacts, asking how COVID maps onto existing disparities within health systems, among health and key workers, as well as low- and high-risk populations (Adey, 2016; Sheller, 2018). Our attention then turns to the meso level, exploring how national health systems are predicated on mobility and the logistical and temporal hurdles that accrue when attempting to mobilise logics of production and transport outside globalisation's pre-negotiated trajectories. Moving on to the macro level, we follow the effects of government mobilisation as they have an impact on international borders, which are sites where the imperative to protect the health and welfare of the population frequently butts up against countervailing impulses rooted in economic arguments and the logic of security and defence. The penultimate section considers how the interaction of these scales – micro, meso and macro – produced a pattern of health inequalities affecting a particular mobile population: migrants. In concluding, we reflect on how this 'mobile assemblage of contingent subjects, enacted contexts and fleeting moments of practice' helps us reconsider what politics and justice in a post-COVID society of moving parts might look like (Sheller, 2018: 20).

Micro level: essential mobilities and health inequalities

In the UK, the lockdown order 'Stay at Home, Protect the NHS, Save Lives' had divergent effects for different communities, casting light on a decade of widening health inequalities (Marmot, 2020). Health inequalities comprise differences in health status, and access to and quality of care and structural determinants of health, for example access to employment and housing (Smith et al., 2016). COVID further exposed health inequalities in UK society, making the marginal and unsafe nature of particular groups' lives more visible, laying bare the links between power and the differential access to and use of health resources. At the local level, these differentials involved particular bodies restricted to particular spaces that have been experiencing poorer health outcomes and inadequate access to health resources for decades (Marmot, 2020). Despite the UK government's assurance that 'we are all in this together', numerous commentators emphasised that, although we may be weathering the same storm, we are not 'all in the same boat' (Glasgow Disability Alliance, 2020). The crisis also inverted the logics of im/mobility, revealing the power differentials that accumulate in a situation where some *essential* things, people and ideas *must* move to save lives, while the majority of *other* things, people and ideas *must not* move to preserve public health (Dobusch and Kreissl, 2020).

Delivery drivers, public transport and warehouse workers, porters and other low-paid employees were suddenly re-labelled as 'key workers'. Indeed, those structurally trapped in poorly paid jobs with low job security and prestige were required to *move* about towns and cities delivering the very services that had locked them into disadvantage by the intersection of class and ethnic inequalities, which produced higher death rates for these workers (Public Health England, 2020; Bhatia, 2020). These 'essential' groups are on the receiving end of significant disparity with respect to material resources, housing, access to green space and private transport. The life-threatening effects of this 'essential mobility' reach deep into the family unit because self-isolation is predicated upon the availability of space. Public health advice stated that if one is potentially infected (because one is moving about in the wider world where the coronavirus is also circulating), at home one should not share a bathroom, bedroom, or kitchen space with family members. Similarly, access to the outdoors and green space – so important for physical and mental health – is limited for those in lower socio-economic groups. Mortality rates in areas of the greatest deprivation were double those in more affluent areas (Public Health England, 2020: 32).

Indeed, the category 'key worker' represented only one example of how the dominant discourse of mobility as desirable and necessary (Urry, 2007) was scrambled and flipped on its head by the COVID lockdown. The prison system, fearing mass contagion, fast tracked prisoners for early release while rough sleepers were pulled off the streets and sequestered in hotels (Pleace, 2020). Neighbours informed on one another if they suspected too much outdoor exercise, while members of the 'kinetic elite' (Cresswell, 2010) – cabinet aides and chief medical officers – continued to travel the length of the country to second homes, breaching guidance to 'Stay at Home' (Bland, 2020; Carrell, 2020). Differential mobilities exposed class divisions and furthered a moral accounting of travel, its rationale and distance. Yet these everyday mobilities and immobilities also imposed starker choices as the means by which that essential movement was channelled: the public transportation systems linking home and work became sites of disease transmission themselves.

In early May, the UK government's public messaging was revised, and England was told to 'Stay Alert'. From a blanket ban enforced by authorities, responsibility shifted to individual members of the public for weighing their gradient of risk and policing their activity accordingly. Yet this daily self-governance also sidestepped questions concerning which bodies could move, be cared for and provide care, and what resources might be utilised to enable this to happen, both locally and internationally. Ultimately, the easing of restrictions heightened temporal and spatial anxieties for at-risk groups dealing with the crisis. 'High-risk' people remained 'shielded' in an enforced 'stillness' (Cresswell, 2012), even as society accelerated around them and equitable access to scarce resources remained an ongoing challenge. (The shielding programme was paused from 1 August with the caveat that it might return as part of future localised lockdowns.)

Risk and protection, access to healthcare and testing, paid work and social welfare are all deeply inflected with questions of mobility and therefore the inequalities and power differentials they produce. In this sense, the crisis and the UK government's variegated response has amplified existing (mobility) inequalities rather than mitigating them, as evidenced most recently by the architecture of the new test-and-trace system. The scheme's initial launch relied heavily on the assumption that test subjects would be highly mobile and capable, in their own cars, to get themselves to drive-through testing centres.

Meso level: national healthcare systems and mobility systems

The Coronavirus Act of 2020 provides a unique window into the UK's governance of the COVID crisis. It grants the government authority to restrict or prohibit public gatherings, suspend public transport systems and infrastructures (including the operation of ports and airports), close businesses, detain suspected carriers of the coronavirus, as well as close childcare and educational facilities, among other capacities. It is an emergency legislation, which grants the government blanket, time-limited decree powers over broad areas of the public, health and economic sectors. On its face, centralised resources and streamlined decision-making were essential tools in coordinating the UK COVID response. Yet as the mobilities literature on crisis notes, the attention of authorities in a crisis tends to narrow towards those 'punctual events' that seemingly require rapid response and timely decision making but which can obscure the 'multiplicity' of the crisis event (Adey and Anderson, 2011) and the 'slow' emergencies (Anderson et al., 2020) that follow in their wake.

One such slower emergency unfolded for disabled people. Despite the seemingly centralised crisis response, the implementation of the Coronavirus Act was in fact largely managed by local authorities, empowering them to limit and suspend services. In the case of disabled people, this differential implementation had dramatic effects: limiting and cancelling social care services to halt the spread of the coronavirus also meant that for many disabled people, mobility within one's own home became significantly restricted (Inclusion London, 2020). This exacerbated the health inequalities and immobility routinely experienced by this population (Goggin and Ellis, 2020) and doubled their morbidity rates (Office for National Statistics 2020).

Years of funding cuts depleted and overturned multiple, integrated layers of infrastructure that would have been ready and waiting for a pandemic event over a decade earlier. For example, in 2013 oversight of public health was reassigned from the independent Health Protection Agency to the smaller Public Health England (PHE) (an agency under the direct control of the Department of Health and Social Care). Local authorities were tasked with taking over the distributed roles of regional PHE observatories and establishing new links with health services. At the time, the reform was criticised for undermining 'pandemic preparedness' (Lawrence et al., 2020; World Health Organization, n.d.). The relocation of PHE's responsibilities also coincided with a decentring of its national prominence: by the time of crisis, the government's Scientific Advisory Group for Emergencies (SAGE) lacked public health expertise and was dominated by modellers and epidemiologists (Scally et al., 2020). Some have suggested this left the UK unable to anticipate and respond to the gaping health inequalities that became evident in COVID infection and death rates (Kelly-Irving, 2020). Thus, as much as the Coronavirus Act formed part of the legal architecture of rapid government mobilisation – in response to a multiplicity of intersecting timelines and contingencies – the government's capacity to act effectively and at scale remained determined by decisions that stretch before and after the particular temporal arc of this crisis (Adey and Anderson, 2011).

While national health systems focus on providing care for static and 'citizen' populations (Kaspar et al., 2019), they are predicated on mobility: both their patients and healthcare workers move between countries, the equipment and life-saving technologies they adopt are sourced from all over the world, and the treatment and triage protocols they deploy are globally co-produced.

The UK's mobilisation of resources and accelerated response faltered beyond the local scale. The successful navigation of this public health crisis required negotiating a complex and dense 'infrastructural backstage' (Graham, 2014) that only comes into full view when globe-spanning medical supply chains, and the established distributions of space-time within which these trajectories of movement are nested, stutter or are disrupted altogether. The issue of testing illustrates the disjunction between the localised, enforced arrestment of society and the global context within which policies were enacted. Over the course of three weeks, beginning on 11 March 2020, the UK government pledged to increase daily testing capacity to 10,000, then to expand this figure to 25,000 (18 March) and finally to reach the figure of 250,000 tests per day (25 March). On 31 March it admitted that its ability to increase testing capacity was being 'hampered' by a global shortage of chemical reagents for the test, and it was only on 2 April that testing surpassed 10,000 people a day. In the midst of this (18 March), the government also announced the purchase of 3.5 million antibody tests and another 17.5 million antibody tests (31 March) when the former tests were found to have too high an error rate.

Over the same period, the UK government was also trying to replenish rapidly dwindling personal protective equipment (PPE) supplies for National Health Service (NHS) staff amid a global shortage, as well as attempting to enlist domestic manufacturers in a 'ventilator challenge' to build 30,000 ventilators that it believed would be needed in a matter of weeks. These issues of procurement illustrate how, at the global and regional level, the channelling, redirecting and repurposing of mobile flows were most responsive to economies of scale (for example procurement arrangements as a single block like the EU rather than as a single state entity) and remain constrained by existing pathways and pre-determined corridors of movement.

Macro level: borders in an im/mobile world

The COVID pandemic has reversed one of the conventional ways of understanding the relationship between crisis and mobility, whereby the mobility of people (refugees and migrants) is produced as a result of an emergency (Adey, 2016). Much as with movement at local levels, international migration, the phenomenon at the heart of the most consequential political struggles of the past decade, largely came to a halt, at least temporarily (Aleinikoff, 2020). Yet those who migrated or fled their countries, and whom the pandemic immobilised at different stages in their journeys, remained. Unlike settled citizens, these migrants were differentially situated vis-à-vis the new immobility regime because although mobility is always a factor in public health, the international border is a particularly fraught site of their interaction. This is complicated by the fact that borders are themselves on the move. According to critical border scholars, it is no longer sufficient to understand borders as fixed divides between jurisdictions. They are, instead, 'a moving barrier, an unmoored legal construct' (Shachar, 2020). Borders have not only become ubiquitous, but they are also frequently located 'wherever selective controls are to be found, such as, for example, health and security checks' (Balibar, 2002: 84).

The work of Foucault alerts us to the modern history of the biopolitical border – the privileged site for the exercise of that state power concerned with the general welfare of the population (biopower). It is a concept that attempts 'to capture the relationship of borders, understood as regulatory instruments, to populations and their movement, security, wealth, and health' (Walters, 2002: 562). In the early 21st century, the regulatory emphasis (particularly in the Global North) was on protecting the security and wealth of populations. This involved curtailing the illicit mobilities of unwanted 'economic migrants' and restricting their asylum rights in the name of security and curbing terrorism. But health was never far from the minds of those actors seeking to heighten the exclusionary function of the border.

For example, in Italy in 2017, as right-wing forces capitalised on the backlash against the mass arrivals of seaborne migrants, 'they bring disease' became an anti-immigrant rallying cry (Greenburgh, 2017). Seaborne migrants do not import dangerous pathogens but they are at risk of communicable disease, due to the violence they experience in transit and unsanitary conditions of transport and temporary accommodation (Prestileo et al., 2015). Arriving migrants are screened for HIV, hepatitis B and C, and tuberculosis, with a positive diagnosis making them eligible for treatment in the Italian healthcare system. But the treatment uptake is limited and uncertain (Prestileo et al., 2015). The well-documented distrust of the healthcare systems of receiving countries (Sargent and Larchanché, 2011) is exacerbated by measures, attempted in many European countries and often resisted by clinicians, that seek to import immigration checks into the clinic (Medact, 2020).

In the UK, health systems were also imbricated in the politics of bordering practices throughout the 2010s (Cassidy, 2019). Particular groups of migrants (including economic migrants) under the Immigration Act of 2014 faced health surcharges and potential exclusion from secondary healthcare under the Immigration Act of 2014 (Department of Health and Social Care, 2020). As the COVID crisis unfolded, the requirement for NHS overseas health and care workers to pay the health surcharge to access the very NHS care they provide touched a political nerve. Negative publicity around this policy compelled the government to eventually drop the surcharge (Proctor, 2020).

The surcharge was a bordering practice in the sense that it discriminated against and stigmatised foreigners working in the NHS. The controversy around it illustrates how bordering practices undermine medical and care recruitment infrastructures, which must secure talent abroad to make up for domestic shortfalls in doctors and nurses. This is a logic that has parallels in other core areas, such as the use of migrant workers in farming or the service sector.

Migrants: healthcare borders in crisis

In this section, we explore the interaction of the micro, meso and macro levels in producing health inequalities in migrant populations. At one level, the bounded nature of healthcare systems has been rendered meaningless by the COVID pandemic itself and the semi-permeable, arbitrary character of borders that must expedite the movement of ideas, technology and resources. At another, the exclusionary and socially captive status of those denied citizenship rights because of immigration or socially marginalised standing have also been reinforced. The construction of migrants as a disease vector emphasises familiar tropes linked to wider discourses surrounding the construction of citizenship and access to its entitlements. Health is a human right that is mediated through citizenship.

Mobility is an increasingly central form of capital in the enactment of this relationship. As Creswell notes: '[T]he capacity to move is central to what it is to be a citizen and, at the same time, the citizen has to be protected from others who move differently – the vagabond or the "alien". Mobility does its work as self and other' (Creswell, 2013: 86). During the pandemic, health advocates have sought to draw attention to the issue of migrant health rights through international declarations and local campaigns focused around the public health imperative to 'leave no-one behind' (International Organisation for Migration, 2020; Lancet Migration, 2020). These declarations speak to the increasing recognition of differences in the entitlement, access and quality of healthcare for migrants at global, national and local levels. They also underscore that entitlement and access are differentially distributed according to one's proximity or distance from citizenship, one's employment status and wider discourses of deservingness, which seem perpetually in flux (Sargent, 2012; Abubakar et al., 2018). Yet in the midst of a pandemic the vulnerabilities of migrant groups should attract particular concern, as evidenced by the case of Singapore – a country once praised for its swift control of the pandemic. The migrant groups that in the first four months of 2020 accounted for the majority of the country's cases were not moving across borders. Rather, infection rates ballooned within the massive foreign worker dormitories on the city's periphery, where Singapore's 200,000-strong army of low-paid service and construction workers are housed 20 to a room and 15 to a toilet (Stack, 2020).

Singapore's example encapsulates the point that protecting the health of the entire population within national borders requires *including* and making *visible* precisely those with limited access to the healthcare system, a recognition that some governments have begun to make. Portugal declared that all migrants with a pending residency application would be treated as residents throughout the crisis, allowing them access to health services, benefits and legal status. Ireland granted undocumented migrants temporary but full access to benefits and healthcare. Saudi Arabia and Qatar also promised free healthcare to the migrant workers on which their economies depend (Reidy, 2020). Yet despite the necessary corrective these temporary 're-borderings' seemingly introduce, they also obscure the long-term limits to healthcare access forged in the last decade whose unintended effects have greatly complicated the governance of this crisis.

In the UK, a 'hostile environment' has been designed to limit the ease of living, working and accessing services for migrants. This involves a range of policy measures and disciplinary instruments across housing, employment, welfare and healthcare systems to limit entitlement and access. As we have already noted, this policy has involved charging for secondary healthcare at the point of delivery (British Medical Association, 2019) and attempts to incorporate healthcare providers into the government's bordering architecture. It has resulted in the outright denial of access to healthcare as well as a documented rise in health issues among refugees and asylum groups (Equality and Human Rights Commission, 2018). It also included proposals for sharing data between the departments of Immigration and Health—a move that was subsequently resisted (Potter, 2018). While exemptions from NHS charges for the diagnosis and treatment of COVID were granted at the start of the crisis (Department of Health and Social Care, 2020), this was neither widely understood nor effective in terms of encouraging people to seek treatment – not least because migrants feared being charged for other treatment and that staff would pass their data to the Home Office, thereby exposing them to potential detention and deportation (Medact, 2020). At the same time, asylum seekers socially distancing in their flats were told to pack their belongings with hours of notice and concentrated in hotel accommodation, where maintaining social distancing was impossible and where reports emerged that access to healthcare had been denied (Santamarina Guerrero, 2020).

At the time of writing (June 2020), infection rates in the UK were declining and the emphasis was shifting to testing and tracing individuals who might have been exposed to the coronavirus: a challenge of identifying and squashing outbreaks before they escalate. Just as in Singapore, it is vital in this effort to identify outbreaks amongst migrant communities. Before COVID, many experts warned that instilling fear in undocumented migrants was detrimental to public health and it remains to be seen how this 'invisible' and excluded population, especially of undocumented migrants, will be picked up on the test-and-trace radar (Kerani and Kwakwa, 2018).

Conclusion

The UK government slogan 'Stay Home, Save Lives, Protect the NHS' illustrates a crisis narrative (Roitman, 2014) that legitimates political decisions and judgements by making certain actions and practices visible and inevitable, while marking others off as invisible and unthinkable. Yet this 'singularity' view of the crisis obscures the multiplicity of decisions at many levels, and within a host of interwoven and interdependent systems, that inhere within and assert themselves before and after a crisis event. The singular goal of 'Protect the NHS' failed to account for the fact that the NHS is a *mobility system* connected to, and dependent upon, a staggering assortment of complex and distantiated systems: chains of circulation weaving together care home systems, international migration systems, medical supply chains, transportation systems and aviation infrastructures. The governance of the pandemic is improvised on the basis of the shifting imperatives of public health, protecting the economy and preserving political power. In the process it reveals the arbitrary and transient nature of the regulatory and infrastructural arrangements underpinning global mobility.

As John Urry (2007) argues, the sheer complexity of space–time coordination and number of moving parts involved exposes these increasingly interdependent networks to significant vulnerability at the best of times. The singularity view renders invisible the 'slow emergency' of austerity programmes and borders across nations in the Global North, exemplified by the UK welfare reform programme of the past decade. The impact of austerity works at multiple spatio-temporal scales: on individual's bodies and minds, communities and the health systems designed to support the nation's health (Marmot, 2020).

Adopting a mobilities approach enables us to interrogate and challenge these singular narratives through an engagement with the complex interconnections between multiple scales and the ways in which these result in differential health im/mobilities (Sheller, 2018). In the COVID context, the mobilities framework has enabled us to think through the exercise of power through the management of bodies by the government's orders to 'Stay at Home, Protect the NHS, Save Lives' in order to limit the transmission of the coronavirus. This approach has enabled us to show how the molecular scale is linked to broader logistics of globalisation, including the provision of supplies to care for people. It also provides a lens through which we challenge pre-pandemic practices around provision and access to healthcare, and previous dogma around 'who counts' in our societies by highlighting dynamics of power that are expressed through shifting im/mobilities of people. In so doing, the mobilities framework offers a means to disrupt centralised responses predicated on static frameworks. The focus on movement enables the articulation of demands for mobility justice, which forms an essential component of any social justice agenda.

References

Abubakar I, Aldridge RW, Devakumar D and Orcutt M (2018) The UCL–Lancet Commission on Migration and Health: the health of a world on the move. *Lancet* 392: 2606–2654.

Adey P (2016) Emergency mobilities. *Mobilities* 11 (1): 32–48.

Adey P and Anderson B (2011) Event and anticipation: UK Civil Contingencies and the space-times of decision. *Environment and Planning A* 43: 2878–2899.

Aleinikoff A (2020) The fragility of the global mobility regime. Retrieved from https://publicseminar.org/2020/05/the-fragility-of-the-global-mobility-regime (accessed 3 June 2020).

Anderson B, Grove K, Rickards L and Kearnes M (2020) Slow emergencies: temporality and the racialized biopolitics of emergency governance. *Progress in Human Geography* 44 (4): 621–639.

Balibar E (2002) *Politics and the Other Scene*. London: Verso.

Bhatia M (2020) COVID-19 and BAME Group in the United Kingdom. *The International Journal of Community and Social Development* 2 (2): 269–272.
Bland A (2020) Dominic Cummings tries to explain when and why of lockdown trip. Retrieved from www.theguardian.com/politics/2020/may/25/dominic-cummings-tries-to-explain-when-and-why-of-lockdown-trip (accessed 6 August 2020).
British Medical Association (2019) *Delayed, Deterred, and Distressed: The Impact of NHS Overseas Charging Regulations on Patients and the Doctors Who Care for Them*. Report. London: British Medical Association.
Carrell S (2020) Scotland's chief medical officer quits over second home row. *The Guardian*, 5 April. Retrieved from www.theguardian.com/uk-news/2020/apr/05/scotland-chief-medical-officer-seen-flouting-lockdown-advice-catherine-calderwood (accessed 6 August 2020).
Cassidy K (2019) Everyday bordering, healthcare and the politics of belonging in contemporary Britain. In: Passi A, Prokkola E, Saarinen J and Zimmerbauer K (eds) *Borderless Worlds for Whom? Ethics, Moralities and Mobilities*. New York: Routledge, pp. 78–92.
Cresswell T (2010) Towards a politics of mobility. *Environment and Planning D: Society and Space* 28: 17–31.
Cresswell T (2012) Mobilities II: still. *Progress in Human Geography* 36 (5): 645–653.
Cresswell T (2013) Citizenship in worlds of mobility. In: Soderstrom O, Ruedin D, Randeria S, D'Amato G and Panese F (eds) *Critical Mobilities*. London: Routledge, pp. 81–100.
Department of Health and Social Care (2020) NHS visitor and migrant cost recovery programme. Retrieved from www.gov.uk/government/collections/nhs-visitor-and-migrant-cost-recovery-programme (accessed 6 August 2020).
Dobusch L and Kreissl K (2020) Privilege and burden of im-/mobility governance: on the reinforcement of inequalities during a pandemic lockdown. *Gender, Work & Organization* 27 (5): 709–716.
Equality and Human Rights Commission (2018) *The Lived Experiences of Access to Healthcare for People Seeking and Refused Asylum*. Research report 122, November. London: Equality and Human Rights Commission.
Glasgow Disability Alliance (2020) Same storm, different boats. Retrieved from https://mailchi.mp/gdaonline/same-storm-different-boats (accessed 1 July 2020).
Goggin G and Ellis K (2020) Disability, communication, and life itself in the COVID-19 pandemic. *Health Sociology Review* 29 (2): 168–176.
Graham S (2014) Disruption. In: Adey P, Bissell D, Hannam K, Merriman P and Sheller M (eds) *The Routledge Handbook of Mobilities*. London: Routledge, pp. 468–471.
Greenburgh R (2017) Italy's echos of fascism as immigrants blamed for disease, rape. Retrieved from https://worldcrunch.com/world-affairs/italy39s-echos-of-fascism-as-immigrants-blamed-for-disease-rape (accessed 12 June 2020).
Inclusion London (2020) *Abandoned, Forgotten and Ignored: The Impact of the Coronavirus Pandemic on Disabled People*. Interim report, June. London: Inclusion London.
International Organisation for Migration (2020) The rights and health of refugees, migrants and stateless must be protected in COVID-19. Retrieved from www.iom.int/news/rights-and-health-refugees-migrants-and-stateless-must-be-protected-covid-19-response (accessed 23 June 2020).
Kaspar H, Walton-Roberts M and Bochaton A (2019) Therapeutic mobilities, *Mobilities* 14 (1): 1–19.
Kelly-Irving M (2020) Health inequalities in a time of pandemic: do we really care? Retrieved from https://researchfrontier.wordpress.com/2020/05/16/health-inequalities-in-times-of-pandemic-do-we-really-care (accessed 23 June 2020).
Kerani RP and Kwakwa HA (2018) Scaring undocumented immigrants is detrimental to public health. *American Journal of Public Health*, 108 (9): 1165–1166.

Lancet Migration (2020) Leaving no one behind in the COVID-19 Pandemic: a call for urgent global action to include migrants and refugees in the COVID-19 response. Retrieved from www.migrationandhealth.org/migration-covid19 (accessed 25 June 2020).

Lawrence F, Garside J, Pegg D, Conn D, Carrel S and Davies H (2020) How a decade of privatisation and cuts exposed England to coronavirus. *The Guardian*, 31 May. Retrieved from www.theguardian.com/world/2020/may/31/how-a-decade-of-privatisation-and-cuts-exposed-england-to-coronavirus (accessed 18 August 2020).

Marmot M (2020) *Health Equity in England: The Marmot Review 10 Years on*. Report, February. London: Health Foundation.

Medact (2020) *Patients Not Passports: Challenging Healthcare Charging in the NHS*. Report. London: Medact. Retrieved from www.medact.org/wp-content/uploads/2020/06/Patients-Not-Passports-Migrants-Access-to-Healthcare-During-the-Coronavirus-Crisis.pdf (accessed 11 December 2020).

Office for National Statistics (2020) Comparisons of all-cause mortality between European countries and regions: January to June 2020. Retrieved from www.ons.gov.uk/peoplepopulationandcommunity/birthsdeathsandmarriages/deaths/articles/comparisonsofallcausemortalitybetweeneuropeancountriesandregions/januarytojune2020 (accessed 11 August 2020).

Pleace N (2020) Homelessness, bad housing, and the virus: a decent home should be every citizen's right. Retrieved from https://blogs.lse.ac.uk/politicsandpolicy/homelessness-and-covid19/ (accessed on 23 June 2020).

Potter JL (2018) Patients not passports: no borders in the NHS. *Justice Power and Resistance* 2 (2): 417–429.

Prestileo T, Di Lorenzo F and Corrao S (2015) Infectious diseases among African irregular migrants in Italy: just an individual problem? *Clinical Social Work and Health Intervention* 2 (5): 45–57.

Proctor K (2020) Johnson forced to drop surcharge for migrant health workers. *The Guardian*, 21 May. Retrieved from www.theguardian.com/world/2020/may/21/johnson-forced-to-drop-nhs-surcharge-for-migrant-health-workers (accessed 6 August 2020).

Public Health England (2020) *COVID-19: Review of Disparities in Risks and Outcomes*. Report, June. London: Public Health England.

Reidy E (2020) Coronavirus: a window of opportunity for action on migration? *The New Humanitarian*, 10 June.

Roitman J (2014) *Anti-Crisis*. Durham, NC: Duke University Press.

Santamarina Guerrero A (2020) Asylum seekers in hotels in Glasgow denied health care by Mears. Retrieved from https://bellacaledonia.org.uk/2020/06/16/asylum-seekers-in-hotels-in-glasgow-denied-health-care-by-mears/ (accessed 20 June 2020).

Sargent C (2012) 'Deservingness' and the politics of health care. *Social Science and Medicine* 74: 855–857.

Sargent C and Larchanché S (2011) Transnational migration and global health: the production and management of risk, illness, and access to care. *Annual Review of Anthropology* 40, 345–361.

Scally G, Jacobson B and Abbasi K (2020) The UK's public health response to covid-19. *British Medical Journal* 369. Retrieved from https://www.bmj.com/content/369/bmj.m1932 (accessed 11 January 2021).

Shachar A (2020) Borders in the time of COVID-19: what the pandemic reveals about the regulation of mobility. Retrieved from https://publicseminar.org/2020/04/borders-in-the-time-of-covid-19 (accessed 12 June 2020).

Sheller M (2018) *Mobility Justice: The Politics of Movement in an Age of Extremes*. London: Verso.

Smith KE, Bambra C and Hill SE (2016) *Health Inequalities: Critical Perspectives*. Oxford: Oxford University Press.

Stack MK (2020) A sudden coronavirus surge brought out Singapore's dark side. *The New York Times*, 20 May.

Urry J (2007) *Mobilities*. Cambridge: Polity.

Walters W (2002) Mapping Schengenland: denaturalizing the border. *Environment and Planning D: Society and Space* 20: 561–580.

World Health Organization (n.d.) Public health preparedness. Retrieved from www.who.int/influenza/preparedness/en/ (accessed 18 August 2020).

4

PHYSICAL ACTIVITY AND BODILY BOUNDARIES IN TIMES OF PANDEMIC

Holly Thorpe, Julie Brice and Marianne Clark

Waking weary from another restless night
Head and heart feeling heavy, I push out
Weaving through quiet neighbourhoods
Towards the beach for fresh air and perspective
Jogging gently over the grass, following the sound of crashing waves
Passing through an open gate
Without thinking, a hand brushes the metal frame
Unwanted touch with bodies before and after
That hand, swinging at my side, burning with new attention
A site of possible contagion
Without sanitiser or wipes in my pocket
Do not touch my face, repeated again and again as I stride.

Bodily rhythms
Feet sinking and lifting from soft sand
Instead of relaxation, new worries creep into familiar movements
A couple walking ahead, a dog running freely
Bounding towards me
Muscles freeze at the possibility of human–animal collision
The dog disobeys the owner's desperate calls
Fur and warmth suddenly pressing against my legs
It all feels too much, turning for home
To wash my clothes and skin
Clean

The physical and mental health benefits of physical activity have been well documented, including in environments of high risk and/or ongoing physical and psychological stress (Stubbs et al., 2017). Recognising the importance of physical activity for health and well-being during the early months of the COVID-19 pandemic, the World Health Organization and many governments encouraged populations to remain physically active, offering various sets of guidelines and recommendations (Chen et al., 2020; Sallis and Pratt, 2020; World Health Organization, 2020). However, while exercise was often encouraged and in many places considered an 'essential activity', options for engagement were increasingly constrained. Commercial fitness centres were closed and many countries also closed parks, beaches and other outdoor recreational facilities, with such closures felt unevenly (Duncan et al., 2020). Important forms of incidental activity accumulated through daily work, shopping and care routines were dramatically diminished (Drake et al., 2020). In other words, people stopped moving in their usual ways.

As a result, our relationships with bodies (our own and those of others) and the spaces and places around us were dramatically altered. For devoted athletes, exercisers and gym-goers, digital spaces became paramount, as a plethora of free offerings (synchronous and asynchronous) emerged from fitness juggernauts such as Kayla Itsines, Les Mills, Strava and Nike, as well as smaller boutique studios and individual instructors (Toffoletti et al., 2020). New leisure and fitness pursuits were also created in backyards, balconies and garages, and in available and allowable public spaces. Sidewalks were soon cluttered with runners and families and children on bikes and scooters. In many countries, daily walks became imperative elements of new daily routines. With the rhythms and routines of physical activity significantly disrupted, many people created alternative movement practices, while others opted for less active lifestyles during periods of quarantine (Garmin, 2020; Sallis and Pratt, 2020).

However, against the backdrop of a pandemic instigated by a virus known to ferociously attack the lungs and other key organs, the rules of engagement had changed. Exercise, once considered a uniformly 'healthy' practice, came to occupy a slippery space in popular and medical discourse (Koren, 2020). Heightened anxieties about viral-laden breath, and moving bodies and their secretions, meant exercise in public spaces was associated with the potential for risk and contagion (Freeman and Eykelbosh, 2020). Suddenly breath and breathing mattered differently, the boundaries of the body thrust into a new light.

In this chapter, we draw upon feminist new materialist theory, particularly the work of Karen Barad, to critically explore new questions about the risks of physically active bodies and the 'trails' of contagion that disperse in and through the ebbs and flows of the natural and built environment. Drawing upon Barad's conceptualisation of bodily boundaries, we explore new ethical considerations and concerns about bodily secretions and exhaled aerosol particles. In so doing, we diffractively read news media releases, scientific reports and public commentaries through our own embodied experiences of physical activity. We then engage new materialist-inspired creative writing in order to evoke vital respondings to some of the entangled relationalities that emerged between moving bodies and broader social and material forces during various stages of COVID. Ultimately, this chapter offers a critical and creative commentary on the new noticings of bodily boundaries in times of pandemic where the body – any and every body – was a site of possible contagion.

New materialism, Barad and bodily boundaries

Over the past five years, scholars working in the context of sport and physical culture have begun to explore the possibilities of new materialisms for '"creatively reimagining" the politics of the moving body as vibrant matter always entrenched within (not beyond) power, politics, knowledge, and discourse' (Newman et al., 2020: 23). Feminist scholars of sport and physical culture have been leading such engagements in the contexts of women's recovery from depression, everyday fitness practices and use of digital technologies (Baxter, 2020; Clark, 2020; Clark and Thorpe, 2020; Fullagar, 2020; Markula, 2019). As such scholars illustrate, feminist new materialisms offer a robust framework for attending to the body's movements, responses and affects, while also acknowledging bodies as socially and culturally produced entities, always 'enmeshed' in broader material-discursive arrangements (see Thorpe et al., 2020). In this essay, we extend such scholarship by thinking and writing specifically with the material-discursive conditions of the moving body during the COVID pandemic.

Drawing upon Niels Bohr's philosophy of physics, Barad's theory of agential realism offers an ethico-onto-epistemological framework that enables an understanding of the productive capacities of *both* discursive and material forces in the creation of social phenomena. Here, matter is relieved from its status as passive substance and imagined as 'agentive, not a fixed essence or property of things' (Barad, 2007: 137). Key to this framework is the concept of intra-action. Agential realism proposes that objects, entities, things, 'do not precede, but rather emerge through, their intra-actions' (Barad, 2007: 33). Importantly, intra-action differs from interaction. Whereas an interaction assumes two independent objects coming together, intra-action focuses on the 'mutual constitution of entangled agencies' (Barad, 2007: 33). Hence, within an agential realist account, 'things don't pre-exist; they are agentially enacted and become determinately bounded and propertied within phenomena' (Barad, 2007: 150). Of particular importance for this chapter are the implications of Barad's agential realism for thinking about corporeal matter and bodily boundaries during COVID.

A long lineage of feminist scholars has been interested in the ways bodies are understood as always 'in the making' (Haraway, 1991: 195) rather than fixed, autonomous entities. Theories such as Donna Haraway's (1991) cyborg theory, Moira Gatens's (1996) imaginary bodies, Nancy Tuana's (2008) viscous porosity, and Samantha Frost's (2016) biocultural creatures all make intellectual overtures towards the ontological inseparability between bodies, machines, environments, affects, and social and scientific knowledges. Feminist geographer Robyn Longhurst (2001) and gender studies and disability scholar Margaret Shildrick (1997), in particular, emphasise the fluid boundaries and messy materiality of the corporeal body. Similarly, Barad looks towards alternative conceptualisations of the body, emphasising that theories which focus exclusively on the human as a singular entity 'miss the crucial point that the very practices by which the differential boundaries of the "human" and "nonhuman" are drawn are always already implicated in particular materializations' (Barad 2003: 824).

Within agential realism, humans are not understood as independent entities but as 'beings in their differential becoming, particular material reconfigurings of the world with shifting boundaries and properties that stabilise and destabilise along with specific material changes' (Barad, 2003: 818). The boundaries of the body are constantly being (re)made depending on the various intra-acting elements within particular material-discursive phenomena. For Barad, 'all bodies, not merely "human" bodies, come to matter through the world's iterative intra-activity – its performativity' (Barad 2007: 152). As we explain in this chapter, the performativities of the world during the COVID crisis worked to further destabilise the body as an 'entity', with many people (not just academics) coming to rethink bodily boundaries. Put simply, the body came to matter differently in the material-discursive conditions of COVID. We now turn to the Baradian-inspired diffractive methodology that facilitated new insights into human movement practices and bodily boundaries in times of a global pandemic.

A diffractive methodology of moving bodies in the COVID crisis

Taking up the ethico-onto-epistemological challenges of new materialisms, scholars are increasingly engaging with Barad's diffractive methodology to 'revitalize the research process' (Bozalek and Zembylas, 2017: 123). As is common in her work, Barad draws upon physical phenomena as metaphor, defining diffraction as the 'way waves combine when they overlap and the apparent bending and spreading out of waves when they encounter an obstruction' (Barad, 2007: 28). There are no binary distinctions made between what is 'old' and 'new' within the diffractive method. Rather, flows of information and knowledge are thought through one another in order to imagine alternative possibilities. We argue that diffraction is not only an apt metaphor, but also a useful methodology in times of pandemic. COVID is a material-discursive context where viral particles are widely dispersed, connecting and colliding with bodies differently, where we are warned of multiple waves of infection, and 'old' and 'new' ways of knowing continue to refract off human and nonhuman bodies in both recognisable and unrecognisable patterns.

According to Bozalek and Zembylas (2017: 123), diffraction provides 'additional affordances through its connection of the discursive and material, with knowledges themselves intelligible to each other in creative and unpredictable ways'. Recognising such potential, scholars across the disciplines have been engaging with diffractive methodologies in a range of ways (Handforth and Taylor, 2016; Lenz Taguchi and Palmer, 2013). Taking inspiration from such works in our efforts to come to new ways of knowing bodily boundaries in times of COVID, we embarked on a Baradian-inspired diffractive process of reading media releases, scientific reports and public commentaries through our own embodied experiences of physical activity.

Over the initial days, weeks, and months of the COVID pandemic, time seemed to blur, but the internet continued to churn, unleashing new information at an impossible pace and dripping with affect – fear, anger, frustration, despair and, eventually, hope. Domestic and international policies moved just as frantically, and scientific studies communicated by both mainstream and social media seemed to offer a whirlwind of contradictory evidence. These knowledges became integrated into our diffractive meaning-making processes.

Running and cycling bodies were said to pose additional risk because aerosols were more widely dispersed through people's noses and mouths as they exercised (Scanlan, 2020; Thoelen, 2020). For example, a computer simulation from a team of Belgian engineers that tracked the 'spread droplets' and 'slipstream' of the exhalations, coughs and sneezes of people while running, walking and cycling went viral. The visual representation of the simulated running bodies shedding a large flume was shared and reposted across various news outlets and social media platforms the world over, with the researchers recommending a distance of 16 feet behind someone walking; 33 feet behind someone running or biking slowly; and 65 feet behind someone biking vigorously (Blocken et al., 2020). The credibility of the research was later questioned by epidemiologists and virologists (Samuel, 2020), but debates continued to rage among exercising communities as to the risks of participating outdoors, as well as the benefits and limitations of wearing a mask while exercising outdoors (Moore, 2020). These were debates that we read avidly across media platforms, and lived and felt through our own moving bodies, while running and walking in our local neighbourhoods in New Zealand and Australia and exercising at home in converted workout spaces.

In the first few weeks of large-scale self-quarantine periods, medical experts also issued public warnings about exercising bodies in public spaces. For example, Australian journalist and medical professional Dr Norman Swan recommended the public 'steer clear' of runners because 'if they invade your personal space, they are flicking whatever secretions they've got' (Scanlan, 2020). Whereas Swan directed his concerns at the breath and sweat of runners, others issued warnings about runners spitting, with concerns that spit not only contains saliva but also sputum from the lungs or drainage from the posterior nasopharynx. In neoliberal societies, exercising bodies are typically celebrated for taking responsibility for individual health, but in the context of COVID, runners and cyclists were seen as a new threat, potentially spreading the virus to others widely as they move. At the same time, many governments continued to remind their populations of the importance of physical activity for their mental health and well-being. For many people, the competing messages around exercising bodies were disorienting and fear inducing, prompting new movement practices and routines.

As feminist scholars of the moving body, we paid particular attention to discussions and debates about bodily secretions (sweat, spit) and exhaled aerosol particles (breath) connecting – intra-acting– with the environment (air, wind, water). We critically engaged with scientific studies documenting the extended radius of dispersion of physically active bodies – panting, puffing and moving with momentum – as well as the responses to such articles in mainstream and social media. As we engaged in physical activity ourselves, we reflected on how this new scientific 'evidence' of transmission and infectious dose impacted our conceptualisation of bodily boundaries, and our movement practices and respondings in navigating other moving bodies in different environmental situations (Shields et al., 2020). In our own communities – in our homes too – we witnessed much debate and contestation over scientific and medical 'warnings', governmental policies (unevenly) restricting outdoor recreation and public responses to, and regulation of, transgressive exercising bodies. Adopting a diffractive methodology, we engaged in an ongoing process of reading (and feeling) the scientific studies, media commentaries and responses, and our own and others' moving bodies, through each other. This was a messy and affective process, and we embraced the intellectual and embodied tensions and confusions that it brought to the fore. Our diffractive methodology was further enabled by an ongoing process of collaborative writing creation. As we discuss below, this creative research process helped us further orient our focus to the materiality of bodily processes, relationships, and entanglements in times of COVID.

Creative representation of entangled bodies in times of contagion

New materialist scholars are increasingly negotiating the challenges of representation that go beyond text, language and the human. Consequently, many are experimenting with different ways to represent their research that account for the materiality of the phenomena under investigation (for example, Fullagar, 2020; Hickey-Moody et al., 2016; Lupton, 2019). In so doing, scholars are taking seriously new materialist critiques of representation and MacLure's (2013: 658) call for approaches that involve creative 'research practices capable of engaging the materiality of language itself'. One approach has been the use of poetry and creative writing in order to disrupt traditional linguist representational patterns and 'bring into view the non-human and human entanglement of agency' (Fullagar, 2020: 181).

As COVID spread around the world, creeping ever closer to home, we, like others working in feminist spaces, turned to the creative possibilities of collaborative writing as a form of sense-making (Abdellatif and Gatto, 2020; Fullagar and Pavlidis, 2020). Specifically, we engaged a post-qualitative-inspired 'poetic inquiry' to support our meaning-making of the materialities of the mysterious and risk-laden pathogens with which we found ourselves living (Fullagar, 2020; Lupton, 2019; St Pierre, 2015). Faced with unprecedented social conditions and intensified concerns and anxieties over the vulnerabilities of one's body, our usual frames for making sense of risk and lived experiences of health or illness seemed insufficient. Embarking on a collaborative writing experiment, we found inspiration in the creative and poetic approaches developed by feminist new materialists focused on health and the body (for example, Fullagar, 2020; Lupton, 2019) for listening to (or con-versing with) the multiplicities of human and nonhuman agents in our material-discursive entanglements.

'Writing-feeling together' became an imperfect but vital effort to make sense of a dramatically altered world, to navigate the unfolding affective atmosphere(s) wrought by COVID (Vannini, 2020) and to think what possible or appropriate responses might be. As we wrote back-and-forth to each other, the social context continued to change rapidly and the pace of our writing intensified in response to these temporal developments. In our collaborative writing we explored these jarring disruptions of our experiences of time, space and matter, as a 'bad flu' became coronavirus, became COVID, became global pandemic, became months of isolation, becoming economic devastation, becoming mental and physical distress, becoming recovery, differently across the world.

As we wrote, sharing our personal, deeply embodied and theoretically informed diffractive readings via multiple digital platforms, we came to new noticings, vital respondings and ethical considerations of bodily boundaries in times of pandemic. In the remainder of this chapter we offer two pieces from our collaborative writing experiment. The first focuses on the socio-material significance of breath and moving bodies. Prior to COVID, sociologists were increasingly recognising the importance of air, breath and breathing as topics deserving critical scholarly attention (Kinga Allen, 2020; Oxley and Russell, 2020). In the context of the COVID pandemic, breath and breathing have taken on new social, cultural, physiological, psychological and material significance (Mbembe, 2020). As Will (2020) writes, '[O]ur current experience of the pandemic is all about breath. The spread of COVID-19 has created risks in the simple act of breathing …'. And as we note above, the materialities of breath are further complicated when people are engaging in physical activity.

Our second creative piece explores the bodily politics of sweat in times of COVID. It builds upon previous (pre-pandemic) sociological literature that has explored the socio-materialities of bodily fluids, as well as contagion, in spaces of indoor fitness and physical activity (Atkinson, 2017; Cahill, 2006; Newman et al., 2016). In the context of COVID, fitness centres have become fraught spaces where people exert themselves and breathe heavily, and where sweaty hands and bodies come into contact with multiple surfaces. A recent survey revealed that 46.7 per cent of global gym members are planning not to return to their local gym because of the heightened risks of contagion, with 36.6 per cent cancelling their memberships (Rizzo, 2020).

Space and time are important in how the moving body comes to matter differently in the material-discursive conditions of pandemic. Our first creative piece explores running bodies in outdoor spaces and the second focuses on indoor spaces of fitness (for example, gyms, fitness studios). Both are written to evoke a sense of time and the ever-changing perceptions and respondings to risk before-during-beyond COVID. Our writing reflects the diffractive process; the experiences shared are refractive composites of our own moving bodies through scientific studies, through media reports, through social media posts and responses, through conversations with colleagues, friends and family.

Breath: moving bodies in outdoor spaces

Pushing out the door
Shoes laced, running away
From the phone, the computer
The screens that relegate with incessant alerts, news
And public announcements

Of a virus
looming
circulating
living
On planes, boats, moving bodies

The light thud of running shoes, connecting with asphalt
Familiar rhythms offering momentary calm
Old routines, new questions
Others sharing the footpaths
Anxieties building as bodies near
Breath suspended as they pass
Waiting to exhale
Then
Inhalation
Nostrils fill with perfume
But not mine
The trail of others' bodies
Noticed anew

Moving alone now, at dawn
Feet continue to pound
Seeking fresh air, sanity, and perspective
Running in the middle of the street
to avoid the risk of encountering others
A cyclist races by
Too close
Disregarding new spatial rules
A cough
Too close
A cloud of unseen particles
My body veers away
Turning for home, deeply
Offended

Muscles craving movement
After weeks inside
Climbing walls
Pulling on shoes, running for the trees
In the cool shade of the forest
Leaping over tree roots and breathing deeply
The trails are tight, but the risk is supposedly less now
No new cases for a few days, signs of progress

As I run, the worries wick away
Leaning into a tight corner

Trees hugging close
Bodies walking on the other side
A startled choreography of avoidance
They clamber up the bank
To escape the trails of breath
To escape the risk of contagion

Sweat: bodily fluids in fitness centres

They say
The virus persists
Alive on surfaces, for days
Determined
Everyday spaces now
Becoming fraught
Risky

A tickle in my throat
A creeping sense of panic
Instructing class warm-up
Hypervisible at the front of the studio
Within minutes a need to wipe my nose
Questioning eyes
'Does she have it?'
I anticipate accusations
'You were abroad?'
Ashamed and nervous
Am I doing the right thing?
Reconfigured social rules
Reimagined ethics
These are the beginnings of
Pandemic times

Gyms closed
Weeks in isolation
Agitations and tensions
Building in bodies
Digital workouts
Queer intimacies
Little squares of screen
Filled with bodies
This strange blurring
Of the public and private

Collectively, flattening the curve
Back to 'normal' soon, perhaps, they tease

But doubts linger
Contagion is still possible
Gyms and fitness studios reopening
Who will return?

Approaching the door,
the familiarity is comforting
But everything is different
hand sanitiser at every turn
New safety notices taped to the walls
Markings on the floor
Sweat glimmers on surfaces
Reaching for the cloth, I hesitate
Trails of contagion visible in new ways
An old friend, coming close
Hesitation

Water fountains, bathroom taps
Workout equipment, yoga mats
Familiar objects hold new meaning
In this space, we share, air, objects
Bodies entangling in new ways
Risk calculations, negotiations
New moral considerations

From the initial emergence of this collaborative project to the culminative stages of writing, the practice of 'being-acting-feeling together' in nonlinear and unfamiliar ways (MacLellan and Talpalaru, 2012: 1), has helped us make meaning of new human and nonhuman entanglements during the extraordinary conditions of a global pandemic. As Lenz Taguchi and Palmer (2013: 639) remind us, at times we need 'others in order to displace and unhinge' our own understandings, and working together with new materialist theory and creative writing processes helped encourage and support an openness (and thus vulnerability) to other ways of knowing the moving body under the rapidly shifting socio-material health conditions of COVID. Writing back and forth across the Tasman ocean through multiple communications platforms and in ways that exceeded our 'usual' academic frames – diffractively thinking our own experiences through each other, all the while reading these through media releases, scientific studies, and social media posts – it could be said that the process of writing together was as 'an experimental feminist praxis of doing collaborative writing [and thinking] differently' (Handforth and Taylor, 2016: 627).

But more than offering us a much-valued safe space to share our thoughts and feelings during an extremely challenging time, our feminist new materialist-inspired collaborative writing experiment prompted vital respondings to our always entangled becoming with other human and nonhuman agents (i.e. a dog on the beach, a cloud of unseen particles, bottles of hand sanitiser, markings on the gym floor). Throughout this collaborative process, the diffractive waves of the COVID pandemic washed up, across and through our moving bodies – each time we went for a walk or run, logged into a digital workout class, or (eventually) re-entered our favourite gym or yoga studio – evoking new affective and ethical relations to our human and nonhuman collaborators, a questioning of bodily boundaries. As feminist scholars of moving bodies entangled in pandemic, new materialist theoretical–inspired creative processes invigorated a new ethics of relation.

Conclusion

In this essay, we drew upon a feminist new materialist theoretical approach, in particular Barad's agential realism, to illustrate how the physically active body prompted new noticings and respondings during COVID quarantine periods. Diffractively reading scientific studies, media commentaries and our own lived experiences through each other, and engaging in an ongoing collaborative creative writing process, we evoked these noticings via examples of 'breath' and 'sweat' in different spaces of physical activity. Through a diffractive analysis of physically active bodies, we highlight some of the 'very practices by which the differential boundaries of the human and the nonhuman are [re]drawn' during a global pandemic (Barad, 2007: 153; brackets added). As well as new noticings of physical boundaries of bodies, we found that in the material-discursive conditions of COVID, the moving body also evoked new ethical and moral boundaries of risk.

Our collaborative poetic inquiry was triggered by new and urgent concerns as to how we might know recent tragic and troubling events differently. Working outside of the confines of the familiar, linear modes of writing, we found alternative spaces for new thoughts and affects that contributed to the messy, entangled, continuously unfolding processes of meaning-making during a global pandemic. As Rosengarten (2020) writes on rethinking breath in the material-discursive conditions of COVID in which scientific thought dominates, we need to find ways to 'appreciate an ongoing creative process that might enable us to become more creative in our response'. For us, our theoretically informed writing practices brought to the fore the Baradian understanding of ethics and response-ability in which we are all (humans and nonhumans) already responsible 'to the others with whom or which we are entangled' (Neimanis, 2018: 393). As feminist scholars of moving bodies living and writing in times of pandemic, such conceptualisations of ethics and reimagining of bodily boundaries seem more urgent than ever.

References

Abdellatif A and Gatto M (2020) It's OK not to be OK: shared reflections from two PhD parents in a time of pandemic. *Gender, Work & Organization* 27 (5): 723–733.

Atkinson M (2017) Ethnoaesthesia: Ashtanga yoga and the sensuality of sweat. In: Sparkes A (ed.) *Seeking the Senses in Physical Culture: Sensuous Scholarship in Action*. New York: Routledge, pp. 63–81.

Barad K (2003) Posthumanist performativity: toward an understanding of how matter comes to matter. *Signs* 28 (3): 801–831.

Barad K (2007) *Meeting the Universe Halfway: Quantum Physics and the Entanglement of Matter and Meaning*. Durham, NC: Duke University Press.

Baxter K (2020) The politics of the gloves: finding meaning in entangled matter. In: Newman J, Thorpe H and Andrews D (eds) *Sport, Physical Culture and the Moving Body: Materialisms, Technologies, and Ecologies*. New Brunswick, NJ: Rutgers University Press, pp. 151–169.

Blocken B, Malizia F, van Druenen T and Marchal T (2020) Towards aerodynamically equivalent COVID19 1.5m social distancing for walking and running. Retrieved from www.urbanphysics.net/COVID19.html (accessed 20 July 2020).

Bozalek V and Zembylas M (2017) Diffraction or reflection? Sketching the contours of two methodologies in educational research. *International Journal of Qualitative Studies in Education* 30 (2): 111–127.

Cahill S (2006) Building bodily boundaries: embodied enactment and experience. In: Waskul D and Vannini P (eds) *Body/Embodiment: Symbolic Interaction and the Sociology of the Body*. New York: Routledge, pp. 69–82.

Chen P, Mao L, Nassis GP, Harmer P, Ainsworth BE and Li F (2020) Coronavirus disease (COVID-19): the need to maintain regular physical activity while taking precautions. *Journal of Sport and Health Science* 9 (July): 103–104.

Clark M and Thorpe H (2020) Towards diffractive ways of knowing women's moving bodies: a Baradian experiment with the Fitbit/motherhood entanglement. *Sociology of Sport* 37 (1): 12–26.

Clark M (2020) Re-imagining the dancing body with and through Barad. In: Newman J, Thorpe H and Andrews D (eds) *Sport, Physical Culture and the Moving Body: Materialisms, Technologies, and Ecologies*. New Brunswick, NJ: Rutgers University Press, pp. 209–228.

Drake T, Docherty A, Weiser T, Yule S, Sheikh A and Harrison E (2020) The effects of physical distancing on population mobility during the COVID-19 pandemic in the UK. *Lancet Digital Health* 2 (August): e385–e387. Retrieved from www.thelancet.com/pdfs/journals/landig/PIIS2589-7500(20)30134–30135.pdf (accessed 15 July 2020).

Duncan P, McIntyre N and Cutler S (2020) Coronavirus park closures hit BAME and poor Londoners most. *The Guardian*, 10 April. Retrieved from www.theguardian.com/uk-news/2020/apr/10/coronavirus-park-closures-hit-bame-and-poor-londoners-most (accessed 10 June 2020).

Freeman S and Eykelbosh A (2020) COVID-19 and outdoor safety: considerations for use of outdoor recreational spaces. Retrieved from https://ncceh.ca/documents/guide/covid-19-and-outdoor-safety-considerations-use-outdoor-recreational-spaces (accessed 12 June 2020).

Frost S (2016) *Biocultural Creatures: Towards a New Theory of the Human*. Durham, NC: Duke University Press.

Fullagar S (2020) Diffracting mind–body relations: feminist materialism and the entanglement of physical culture in women's recovery from depression. In: Newman J, Thorpe H and Andrews D (eds) *Sport, Physical Culture and the Moving Body: Materialisms, Technologies and Ecologies*. New Brunswick, NJ: Rutgers University Press, pp. 170–192.

Fullagar S and Pavlidis A (2020) Thinking through the disruptive effects and affects of the coronavirus with feminist new materialism. *Leisure Sciences*. Epub ahead of print.

Garmin (2020) The effect of the global pandemic on active lifestyles. Retrieved from www.garmin.com/en-US/blog/general/the-effect-of-the-global-pandemic-on-active-lifestyles (accessed 5 June 2020).

Gatens M (1996) *Imaginary Bodies: Ethics, Power and Corporeality*. London: Routledge.

Handforth R and Taylor CA (2016) Doing academic writing differently: A feminist bricolage. *Gender and Education* 28 (5): 627–643.
Haraway D (1991) *Simians, Cyborgs, and Women: The Reinvention of Nature*. New York: Routledge.
Hickey-Moody A, Palmer H and Sayers E (2016) Diffractive pedagogies: dancing across new materialist imaginaries. *Gender and Education* 28 (2): 213–229.
Kinga Allen I (2020) Thinking with a feminist political ecology of air-and-breathing bodies. *Body and Society* 26 (2): 79–105.
Koren M (2020) The healthiest way to sweat out a pandemic. *The Atlantic*, 18 March. Retrieved from www.theatlantic.com/health/archive/2020/03/coronavirus-gyms-exercise-social-distancing/608278 (accessed 2 June 2020).
Lenz Taguchi H and Palmer A (2013) A more 'liveable' school? A diffractive analysis of the performative enactments of girls' ill-/well-being with(in) school environments. *Gender and Education* 25 (6): 671–687.
Lupton D (2019) 'Things that matter': poetic inquiry and more-than-human health literacy. *Qualitative Research in Sport, Exercise and Health*. Epub ahead of print.
Longhurst R (2001) *Bodies: Exploring Fluid Boundaries*. New York: Routledge.
MacLellan M and Talpalaru M (2012) Editors' introduction. *Reviews in Cultural Theory* 2 (3): 1–5.
MacLure M (2013) Researching without representation? Language and materiality in post-qualitative methodology. *International Journal of Qualitative Studies in Education* 26 (6): 658–667.
Markula P (2019) What is new about new materialism for sport sociology? Reflections on body, movement, and culture. *Sociology of Sport Sociology* 36 (1): 1–11.
Mbembe A (2020) The universal right to breathe. *Critical Inquiry*, 13 April. Retrieved from https://critinq.wordpress.com/2020/04/13/the-universal-right-to-breath (accessed 20 July 2020).
Moore P (2020) Should I wear a mask when I'm exercising outside? *The Guardian*, 8 May. Retrieved from www.theguardian.com/us-news/2020/may/08/coronavirus-face-mask-exercise-outside (accessed 4 June 2020).
Neimanis A (2018) Nature represents itself: bibliophilia in a changing climate. In: Kirby V (ed.) *What if Culture was Nature All Along?* Edinburgh: Edinburgh University Press, pp. 179–198.
Newman J, Shields R and McLeod C (2016) The MRSA epidemic and/as fluid biopolitics. *Body and Society* 22 (4): 155–184.
Newman J, Thorpe H and Andrews D (eds) (2020) *Sport, Physical Culture and the Moving Body: Materialisms, Technologies, and Ecologies*. New Brunswick, NJ: Rutgers University Press.
Oxley R and Russell A (2020) Interdisciplinary perspectives on breath, body and world. *Body and Society* 26 (2): 3–29.
Rizzo N (2020) Gyms reopening: 46.67% of members won't return (study). Retrieved from https://runrepeat.com/gyms-reopening-coronavirus (accessed 8 June 2020).
Rosengarten M (2020) The challenge of breath: toward an 'after' COVID-19. *Social Anthropology*. Epub ahead of print.
Samuel S (2020) Why you're unlikely to get the coronavirus from runners or cyclists. Retrieved from www.vox.com/future-perfect/2020/4/24/21233226/coronavirus-runners-cyclists-airborne-infectious-dose (accessed 12 June 2020).
Scanlan R (2020) Doctor warns to 'steer clear' of runners. *NZ Herald*, 1 April. Retrieved from www.nzherald.co.nz/lifestyle/news/article.cfm?c_id=6&objectid=12321647 (accessed 25 May 2020).
Sallis JF and Pratt M (2020) A call to action: physical activity and COVID-19. Retrieved from www.exerciseismedicine.org/support_page.php/stories/?b=896 (accessed 2 June 2020).

Sallis JF, Adlakha D, Oyeyemi A and Salvo D (2020) An international physical activity and public health research agenda to inform COVID-19 policies and practices. *Journal of Sport and Health Science* 9 (4): 328–334.

Shields R, Schillmeier M, Lloyd J and van Loon J (2020) 6 feet apart: spaces and cultures of quarantine. *Space and Culture* 23 (3): 216–220.

Shildrick M. (1997) *Leaky Bodies and Boundaries: Feminism, Postmodernism and (Bio)ethics*. New York: Routledge.

St Pierre E (2015) Practice for the 'new' in the new empiricisms, the new materialisms and post qualitative inquiry. In: Denzin N (ed.) *Qualitative Inquiry and the Politics of Research*. London: Routledge, pp. 75–96.

Stubbs B, Koyanagi A, Hallgren M, Firth J, Richards J, Schuch F, Rosenbaum S, Mugisha J, Veronese N, Lahti J and Vancampfort D (2017) Physical activity and anxiety: a perspective from the World Health Survey. *Journal of Affective Disorders*, 208 (January): 545–552.

Thoelen J (2020) Belgian-Dutch study: Why in times of COVID-19 you should not walk/run/bike close behind each other. Retrieved from https://medium.com/@jurgenthoelen/belgian-dutch-study-why-in-times-of-covid-19-you-can-not-walk-run-bike-close-to-each-other-a5df19c77d08 (accessed 5 June 2020).

Thorpe H, Brice J and Clark M (2020). *Feminist New Materialisms, Sport and Fitness: A Lively Entanglement*. Basingstoke: Palgrave Macmillan.

Toffoletti K, Pavlidis A, Thorpe H and Olive R (2020) Working out at home works for women – so well they might not go back to gyms. *The Conversation*, 26 May. Retrieved from https://theconversation.com/working-out-at-home-works-for-women-so-well-they-might-not-go-back-to-gyms-138111 (accessed 2 June 2020).

Tuana N (2008) Viscous porosity: witnessing Katrina. In: Alaimo S and Hekman S (eds) *Material Feminisms*. Bloomington, IN: Indiana University Press, pp. 188–213.

Tupekci Z (2020) Keep the parks open. *The Atlantic*, 7 April. Retrieved from www.theatlantic.com/health/archive/2020/04/closing-parks-ineffective-pandemic-theater/609580 (accessed 2 June 2020).

Vannini P (2020) COVID-19 as atmospheric dis-ease: attuning into ordinary effects of collective quarantine and isolation. *Space and Culture* 23 (3): 269–273.

Will C (2020) 'And breathe…'? The sociology of health and illness in COVID-19 time. *Sociology of Health and Illness* 42 (5): 967–971.

World Health Organization (2020) Be active during COVID-19. Retrieved from www.who.int/emergencies/diseases/novel-coronavirus-2019/question-and-answers-hub/q-a-detail/be-active-during-covid-19 (accessed 3 June 2020).

5

CITY FLOWS DURING PANDEMICS

Zooming in on windows

Olimpia Mosteanu

> Day-to-day reality, the life we live, is also a fleshy affair. A matter of chairs and tables, food and air, machines and blood. Of bodies.
>
> *(Mol, 2002: 27)*

Zooming in

As an immigrant, windows have welcomed me time and again to new ways of living, reminding me that others are calling my adoptive neighbourhoods their home. As an urbanist, windows fascinate me because they are caught up in a series of dichotomies that posit what is inside against the outside, the intimate against the public, home against street, stability against unpredictability. As a photographer, snapping a quick photograph of someone's window is sign of my positionality, which allows me to engage in this activity without having people stop me to question my motives. For these reasons, by the time the COVID-19 lockdown measures had been imposed in the United Kingdom (in March 2020), I had already compiled a wide-ranging digital archive of hundreds of photographs of windows taken in London and elsewhere.

This chapter examines the role of windows in supporting city dwellers' wellbeing during these times of physical distancing, self-isolation and quarantine. I explore some of the ways in which windows not only mediate our interactions with the world around us but also actively participate in our everyday lives, especially at a time when outdoors activities are restricted because of the pandemic. I approach this analysis from a photographic angle, working with and against the digital archive I have compiled to inquire into more-than-representational dimensions of people's lived experiences. I commence by bringing attention to the role of photography in capturing these dimensions, and consider how this type of photographic enquiry can benefit qualitative research focused on the lived experience of place at a time when in-person methods are no longer an option. I then 'problematise' (Rabinow, 2009) the window and position this chapter within the scholarship about the role played by nonhumans in the lifeworld. This is followed by an exploration of some of the ways in which windows not only mediate our interactions with the world around us but also actively participate in our everyday lives, especially during moments of lockdown and quarantine. Finally, I consider how photographs of windows gesture towards the layered experiences of space and place, as well as the presence and absence of affect and memory.

Urban flows through photographs

In the words of Bourdieu (1990), photography always portrays and betrays the embodied dispositions of the person holding the camera. In the case of COVID lockdown experiences, photographs can easily obscure who can look inside the home, the positionality of the photographer. Who can safely stop and take photos without being seen as a threat by neighbours? Who can move from neighbourhood to neighbourhood, trying to go unnoticed in a variety of socioeconomic contexts? Figure 5.1 brings attention to this very observation: when zooming in on windows, the person holding the camera remains invisible, yet it is this absence that

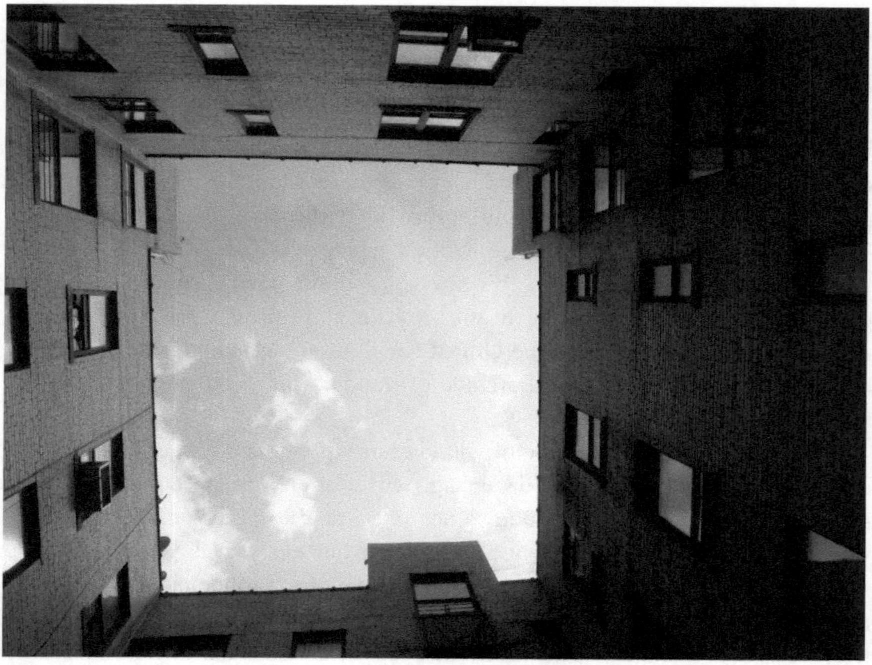

FIGURE 5.1 Zooming in on windows (New York City, 2017)
Source: Olimpia Mosteanu

shapes the photograph and brings the world around into new focus. This photograph also illustrates some other limitations of zooming in on windows, such as the fact the windows of ground floor and first floor homes are easier to capture by the camera, and it highlights the very materiality of windows – their different sizes, shapes and location – which is at the centre of this chapter.

Photographs are tools for producing the city, not only for documenting it. The photographs I include in this visual ethnographic project are not mere representations of city flows. They also reveal particular ways of cataloguing, mapping, and imagining cities, homes and our positions within them. The photographed windows thus disclose as much as they hide about everyday city life. This project nonetheless attempts to remind us that our home in the city is an always-changing artifact that is collaboratively produced by human and nonhuman bodies; in this sense home is a 'more-than-human-assemblage' (Bennett, 2010; Whatmore, 2006) of sorts. This visual ethnography requires us to be attentive to how the photographs surface their own 'conditions of … historical possibility … and the … grid of power that [moulds] and [orders] the physical landscape' (Back, 2009: 477–478). I have worked with photographs bearing in mind that they are tools for producing the home and not only portraying it.

In this chapter, I have approached the research subject from a photographic angle, working with and against the digital archive I have compiled to inquire into more-than-representational dimensions of people's lived experiences. As social researchers are required to replace traditional interactive methods with other means of carrying out place-based research during a pandemic, photo elicitation can add strong visual dimensions to the research design. Photo elicitation is a qualitative research method that, in its most common form, uses photographs taken by research participants to stimulate additional engagement and insight from them. Photographs of places inside the home and of local areas can elicit participants' layered experiences of the physical environment in which they live. Sometimes, they are also able to inform the researcher about experiences that often research participants themselves do not think about, such as how people move in their surroundings, how people instinctively avoid certain spaces because they do not feel entitled to occupy them, the role of daily routines, and so on.

I argue that this enquiry is even more relevant now, given the role nonhumans have played in supporting city dwellers' wellbeing during these times of physical distancing, self-isolation and quarantine. The same is true of the visual methodologies. I hope to show that photography can offer one possible practical, responsive and, hopefully, sensible approach to the study of the social life of places during a pandemic. This approach could help social researchers better understand the social networks, infrastructures, and other aspects of the built environment people rely on and value in their local areas, especially during pandemics. These sometimes go unnoticed to people themselves in their daily lives because they are taken for granted, but they become visible as soon as the everyday order is disrupted. Visual methodologies that carefully consider the materiality of more-than-human assemblages can not only engage the impact of these disruptions but also document and problematise the relationships and practices that have been slowly emerging.

Problematising the window

Outside pandemics, or during what some have started to refer as 'normal times', windows play an important role in safeguarding the borders of home, while also providing access to the city. There are numerous studies showing that natural light and indoor air quality contribute to increased physical and mental health (Sundell et al., 2011; Connellan et al., 2013). Windows bind homes to the street and household routines to the vibrancy of the city, supporting the flow of urban life. They make it impossible for our homes to appear as self-contained bodies, as they connect us across streets or courtyards with other urban forms. Windows sometimes seem to bring houses closer to one another, thus binding the cityscape more tightly together. In other cases, when windows reveal a world completely out of reach for the outsider, they stretch the fabric of the city to its limits, imposing additional material and symbolic distances on city dwellers. Because they bind the home to the outside world, windows direct the life inside towards the outside.

Yet, during my walks in the first few weeks of lockdown in London, I noted that windows started to play unexpected roles. Unlike 'normal times' windows, it seemed as if, during the lockdown, windows were trying to draw in passers-by, to engage them. Figure 5.2 shows some of the different ways in which dwellers were

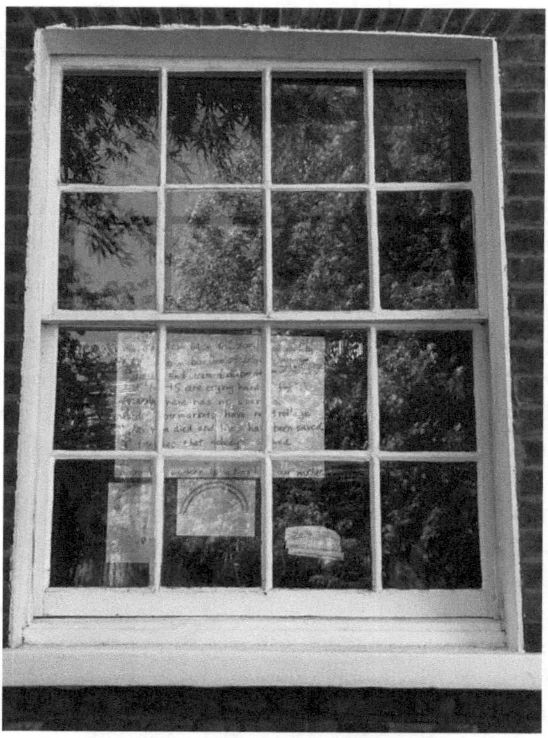

FIGURE 5.2 In the first weeks of the lockdown, windows started to speak (London, May 2020)
Source: Olimpia Mosteanu

starting to communicate with passers-by – through rainbow drawings, which spread across Europe after becoming popular in early March during the lockdown in Italy (Otte, 2020), hopeful written messages and children's drawings. Taken together, these messages were starting to create a different type of city flow, one that was joining homes, windows, streets, dwellers, and affective forces together, making people and homes visible to each other in a different way. All of a sudden, windows directed the life outside towards the inside.

As other city flows came to a halt, it appeared that windows became a way for the city to speak to itself and about itself. In the absence of gardens or balconies, windows seemed to have become the place to take the pulse of the neighbourhood. This realisation made me even more interested in the work windows do to make home possible, especially under duress. As the COVID lockdown put pressure on homes, windows seemed to fulfil a new role in keeping some of the city dwellers grounded in the city. As the lockdown continued, an analysis of the role played by windows during pandemics appeared to me as more and more important.

Windows in more-than-human assemblages

I started thinking about this chapter in early April 2020, when the world of social research came to a halt due to the COVID crisis. Since then, I have tried to understand how social research can continue responsibly and responsively under the fast-changing circumstances of pandemics. In addition to having to address new risks and limitations, social research has to be designed with flexibility and an open mind, given the evolving impact COVID is having on urban flows and the changing governmental responses to it. As with other epidemics and pandemics, COVID has also brought research into particular topics to a halt as new priorities and concerns have been emerging (Roy et al., 2020; Van Loon, 2005). Yet, as Bhan et al. (2020) compellingly argue, it remains essential to problematise these emerging matters of concern and consider how they are entangled with older forms of 'distancing and exclusion'.

The role of nonhumans in the making of homes has gained increased attention in the last few years (Soaita and McKee, 2019), drawing on more-than-human approaches (Bennett, 2010; Ingold, 2007; Whatmore, 2006). This chapter builds on this scholarship by reconsidering the role played by nonhumans in everyday life and rejecting the agency/structure dichotomy. I pay close attention to interactions between various humans and nonhumans (such as windows, rainbow drawings, children's sketches, among others) and seek to find a way to understand their entanglement in a world they created together. This approach to more-than-human assemblages problematises the relationships between humans and nonhumans by carefully examining the intimate involvement of bodies, places and affect. Whatmore (2006) argues that more-than-human geographies amplify (inter)corporeality, as these bring attention not just to human corporeality but to the interconnectedness of human and nonhuman bodies, to the fluidity of bodies. Likewise, Bennett (2004: 365) writes, 'humans are always in composition with nonhumanity, never outside of a sticky web of connections or an ecology [of matter]'.

Following these approaches to more-than-human assemblages, I chart the emerging relationships involved in the everyday production of home through windows. Home does not appear here as a container of relationships between human bodies and things. This visual ethnography claims that, during lockdown, home has emerged out the practical engagement of human and nonhumans that put windows at its centre, at least for a while. The quotation that introduces this chapter, taken from Mol's (2002) ethnography of patients with atherosclerosis, captures neatly the crux of the more-than-human approaches I have drawn on, by directing attention to the fact that everyday life is the making of a wide range of bodies – 'a fleshy affair' that allows us to observe what corporeality is and how it binds humans and nonhumans together.

All things considered, home is always a more-than-human assemblage. The home, like the city itself, is multiple, fragmented and connected to other wider regional and international urban process. It is produced relationally in and through dwelling/knowing practices that include everyday routines such as making and consuming meals, as well as routines that have emerged under duress, during lockdown, which have included painting windows or decorating them with friendly teddy bears (see Figures 5.3 and 5.4). In this respect, I concur with Ingold (2000: 156), who argues that 'the world continually comes into being

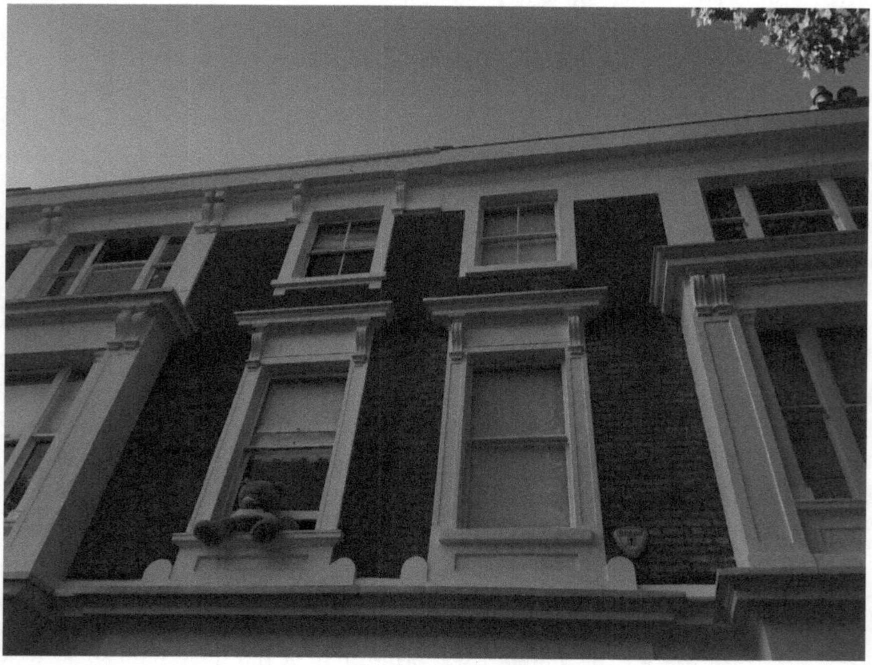

FIGURE 5.3 Understanding city flows during lockdown by making nonhuman bodies legible (London, June 2020)
Source: Olimpia Mosteanu

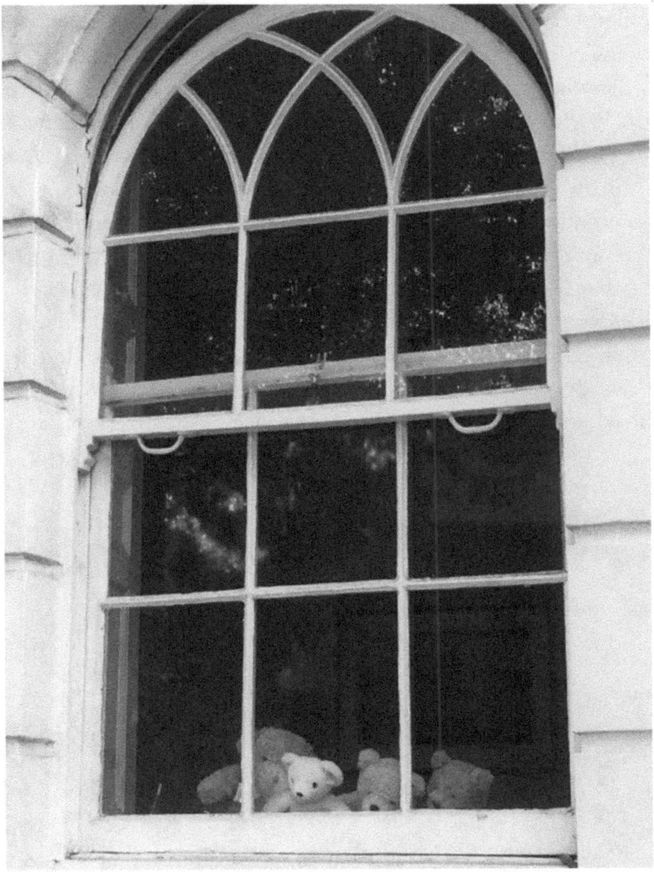

FIGURE 5.4 Communicating bodies (London, June 2020)
Source: Olimpia Mosteanu

around the inhabitant and its manifold constituents through their incorporation into a regular pattern of live activity'. As the next two sections show, we can start to understand some of the city flows that have emerged during lockdown by examining more-than-human assemblages.

Shaping the experience of home: windows in London during lockdown

During the UK lockdown, windows have played a central role in coping strategies, alongside other nonhumans such as digital technologies. As Figures 5.3 and 5.4 show, some dwellers have packed their windows with teddy bears that seemed to wave at the world outside the home, comforting passers-by while creating a channel of communication between home and the city. In this sense, these photographs illustrate the effort of making the home engage the outside world. The teddy bear captured in Figure 5.3 even wears a face covering. It attracted quite a few looks and made many passers-by stop and smile (I spent some time watching it myself and even managed to chat with its owner, who told me that a lot of children waved back at the teddy bear). The 'family' of bears pictured in Figure 5.4 was similarly effective and perhaps more poignant in how it chose to communicate care and togetherness. These more-than-human assemblages have brought together homes, streets, windows, teddy bears but also emotions and memories. In so doing, they have bridged the space of the home and the outside. These observations seem to support Bennett's (2010: 21) claim that 'bodies enhance their power in or as a heterogenous assemblage'.

As we have seen in the photographs, many people in London have filled their windows with drawings and rainbow paintings. Other dwellers chose to dress their windows with messages of support for key workers, their local neighbourhood or the National Health Service (NHS). As Figure 5.5 shows,

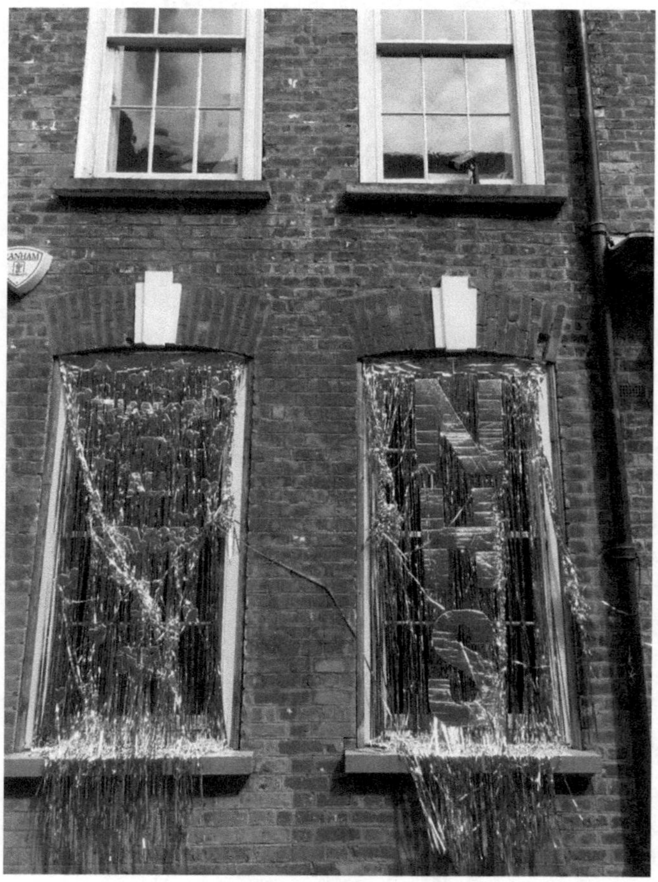

FIGURE 5.5 Can the nonhuman speak? (London, April 2020)
Source: Olimpia Mosteanu

when included in more-than-human assemblages, windows can certainly speak. They can draw attention to issues of concern such as those that have surrounded the NHS and key workers throughout the lockdown (Scambler, 2020). As was the case with the photographs discussed above, neither the dwellers nor the NHS-adorned windows spoke directly to passers-by. The acts of communication are achieved through the assemblage that brings together windows, dwellers, yellow cellophane, as well as feelings of safety, anxiety and the need for dialogue.

Windows, just like digital technologies, helped the home stay connected. In different ways, both have enabled physically distanced social contact and established new regimes of observability (Hine, 2020). Windows, however, have also had the opposite effect from digital technologies on everyday routines in the home: if smart technologies have provided for a targeted but disembodied form of communication during lockdown, windows allowed dwellers to reach out to the larger world outside the home while allowing for safe, physical engagement. By engaging with the window – either by painting it, decorating it or filling it with messages – dwellers have engaged the world outside directly.

The division between public and domestic spaces has been contested by a number of scholars (Grosz, 1995; Martella and Enia, 2020; Perec, 1997) but I would like to argue that, during lockdown, this separation has become even less tenable. Lockdown and physical distancing measures have posited public space as risky and home as a safe environment that protected individuals and public health. Yet some scholars (Brickell, 2020; Gurney, 2020) have questioned whether, from a mental health perspective, home can be thought of as a safe, domestic environment, given the emerging pressures on inhabitants and the risk of family violence. For those working from home, work and work-related routines have taken over intimate quarters. Home schooling has brought public eyes and unexpected surveillance routines into the private realm as well.

I believe, however, that it is misleading to think that it is only working-from-home practices, digital technologies and their regimes of observability, and home schooling that have brought public routines into the home. As I have shown above, during lockdown, as many people have experienced a loss of physical contact, windows have brought the outdoors into the space of the home. Windows have allowed the home to extend itself into the outdoors, to become larger by incorporating, safely, public space. This extension of the space of home into the street, the sidewalk, the parking lot or the empty space between adjacent buildings has been particularly important for homes without access to balconies or gardens.

Certainly not all windows have expanded the home during lockdown, but some have. As I have noted above, windows have not only mediated human interactions with the world around but have also actively participated in them by stabilising emerging forms of interaction with the world outside. By seeing the window as an active agent and not as a passive thing or a household object, we can more easily grasp its material and symbolic affordances: in this case how the window makes possible certain practices of making a home under duress. Human and nonhuman bodies together made life possible during lockdown, and windows played a key role in shaping affect, memory and social interaction as part of more-than-human assemblages. In the absence of 'normal' city flows that bind the home to the city, windows have allowed homes and their dwellers to stay connected, creating a new affective landscape around them.

There is yet another way in which windows played a role in both keeping people connected and allowing the home to extend itself into the outdoors: namely by letting smells and sounds inside the home. Neighbours cooking, singing, playing music and, in the UK, clapping on Thursdays for key workers have shaped the experience of the home and given new meanings to the city during lockdown. As Figure 5.6 illustrates, during lockdown windows have welcomed a wide range of exchanges with the world; they have allowed the city to enter the home and allowed the home to project itself outside into the city. It is important to note that all of these experiences have had a temporal dimension, as they have come into play at a particular moment during the

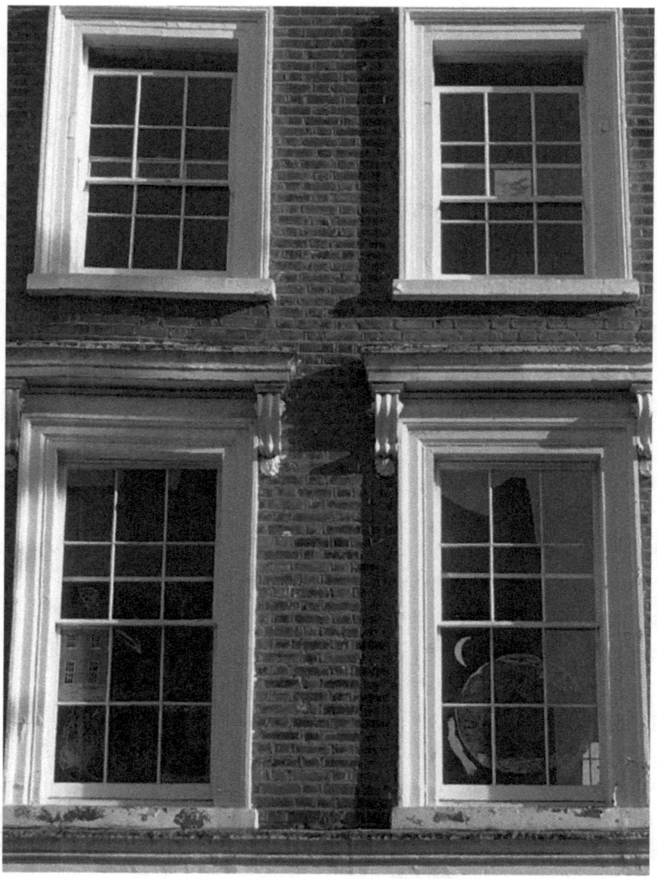

FIGURE 5.6 Window as synecdoche (London, May 2020)
Source: Olimpia Mosteanu

pandemic – think about the communal singing in Italy or the clapping for key workers in the UK – and have evolved over time as people's relationships to the pandemic have shifted. Still, in this collective engagement in practice, these more-than-human assemblages have stitched together the lifeworld. This has been achieved by nonhumans coming together with humans. They have not been not acting alone or separate from each other, but in assemblages.

Windows have shown a capacity to change, to become a different kind of agent. This is why it is so important to think of windows as part of more-than-human assemblages, not as things that are separate from human bodies. Etymologically, a 'thing' signifies a gathering of people. Yet, in most cases, nowadays it means a bounded nonhuman object, which is characterised by inertia. In his recent work, Ingold tries to portray this by pointing out that they are 'knots' of lines along which movement occurs:

> After all, what is a thing, or indeed a person, if not a tying together of the lines – the paths of growth and movement – of all the many constituents gathered there? Originally, 'thing' meant a gathering of people, and a place where they would meet to resolve their affairs. As the derivation of the word suggests, every thing is a parliament of lines.
>
> *(Ingold, 2007: 5)*

Windows bearing messages of support for the NHS and key workers or windows decorated with rainbow drawings and teddy bears are such 'knots of lines' along which movement have occurred during lockdown. These 'parliament of lines' or assemblages have directed the emerging city flows I have outlined above. These knots of lines have made possible for timely acts of communication, care and togetherness to unfold between the city and its homes.

At the same time, the window can also be a lens into understanding the impact of the COVID pandemic on everyday life in relation to social class. It is important to ask how windows spatialise class by offering a differential access to daylight and by affecting air quality and mental health. It is as important to ask what types of dwellings are still designed without access to balconies or windows. For some people, home is part of an infrastructure of care; for others, home plays a significant role in hiding domestic violence (Brickell, 2012, 2020; Gurney, 2020). As such, windows do not always provide clear views into or outside the house, which makes the role of window coverings (curtains, blinds) different from the instances I have discussed above. In hiding such acts of domestic violence, windows retain their active, agential role but the more-than-human assemblage they form is not directed towards supporting acts of exchange and togetherness between the city and home.

If indeed windows have played a role in keeping people connected and in allowing the home to merge with the outdoors, thus supporting physical and mental health, what has the impact of windowless homes been on everyday routines during the COVID pandemic? If windows have actively participated in reminding people that their home is still part of a larger structure, how has the lack of windows impacted the experience of the city for those living in windowless homes (for instance, the experiences of residents in some of England's substandard office-to-residential conversions; see Clifford et al., 2018)? None of these questions can be answered without taking into account wider socioeconomic factors, but it is important to keep in mind that by zooming in on windows I have captured a very limited, however layered, experience of space and place.

The window as synecdoche

In focusing on windows in this chapter, I have directed attention to a particular type of nonhuman that has played a role in supporting the lifeworld during lockdown. The use of photographs has made possible a reflection on the everyday life in the home, which is seen through a variety of practices that relied on windows. During lockdown, windows have been keeping or preserving the reality of a present always-in-the making. They have brought together and maintained people's hopes, fears and everyday thoughts.

In this sense, during lockdown, windows have not only been an extension of the home into the outdoors but also an overflowing of the past into the future, a way of connecting the past to an uncertain future. Windows have held together the home by offering access to fresh air, sunlight and a view to the outside of the home, including of the built and natural landscapes and of other people and living things. In this way, windows have helped in creating a more comfortable present. In cities around the world, windows have also become a communicative medium used by dwellers to dialogue with other people outside the household. They have acted as a reminder of the struggle for a common future and the comforting memory of city flows, and of a moment when we and others cohabited the city together.

Windows, thus, have overflowed temporally by tying human bodies and their homes into wider relationships and urban processes in which no dweller is alone or isolated. They have grounded practices through which the city has become legible again during lockdown. Just as importantly, windows have made possible forms of engagement with more-than-human bodies which, in turn, have constituted the very modalities through which new, meaningful ways of living have been supported. Has this been a story of resilience or adaptability of homes? Perhaps. But it could have also just been a story of the home as a more-than-human assemblage, which has expanded in new ways as a result of new pressures, routines and expectations.

On the one hand, the photographed windows have spun a narrative about the life inside. On the other hand, they have highlighted new ways of being with others while remaining physically distant. Windows have played a key role in grounding the home in the city by supporting emerging city flows during the COVID pandemic. The photographs have captured how an emerging home-in-the-city has been reclaimed materially and symbolically. The photographs have captured the capacity of nonhumans to inhabit an emerging dwelling space alongside humans. At a time riddled with anxiety and uncertainty, place-based research designs need to remain sufficiently flexible in order to accommodate the shifting needs and burdens placed on individuals, neighbourhoods and the research community itself. Perhaps this could be a time when scholars across disciplines experiment together with forms of co-producing knowledge in a pursuit of a research process based on dialogue and exchange of experiences.

References

Back L (2009) Portrayal and betrayal: Bourdieu, photography and sociological life. *Sociological Review* 57 (3): 471–490.

Bennett J (2004) The force of things: steps toward an ecology of matter. *Political Theory* 32 (3): 347–372.

Bennett J (2010) *Vibrant Matter: A Political Ecology of Things*. Durham, NC: Duke University Press.

Bhan G, Caldeira T, Gillespie K and Simone A (2020) The pandemic, southern urbanisms and collective life. Retrieved from www.societyandspace.org/articles/the-pandemic-southern-urbanisms-and-collective-life (accessed 25 August 2020).

Bourdieu P (1990) *Photography: A Middle-Brow Art*. Cambridge: Polity Press.

Brickell K (2012) 'Mapping' and 'doing' critical geographies of home. *Progress in Human Geography* 36 (2): 225–244.

Brickell K (2020) Stay home, stay safe? A political geography of home in Covid-times. Retrieved from https://blog.geographydirections.com/2020/07/08/stay-home-stay-safe-a-political-geography-of-home-in-covid-times/?utm_source=Twitter&utm_medium=social&utm_campaign=SocialSignIn (accessed 22 July 2020).

Butler J (1990) *Gender Trouble: Feminism and the Subversion of Identity*. New York: Routledge.

Clifford B, Ferm J, Livingstone N and Canelas P (2018) Assessing the impacts of extending permitted development rights to office-to-residential change of use in England. Retrieved from www.rics.org/globalassets/rics-website/media/knowledge/research/research-reports/assessing-the-impacts-of-extending-permitted-development-rights-to-office-to-residential-change-of-use-in-england-rics.pdf (accessed 25 August 2020).

Connellan K, Gaardboe M, Riggs D, Due C, Reinschmidt A and Mustillo L (2013) Stressed spaces: mental health and architecture. *HERD: Health Environments Research & Design Journal* 6 (4): 127–168.

Grosz E (1994) *Volatile Bodies: Toward a Corporeal Feminism*. Indianapolis, IN: Indiana University Press.

Grosz E (1995) Bodies-cities. In: Grosz E, *Space, Time, and Perversion: Essays on the Politics of Bodies*. New York: Routledge, pp. 103–110.

Gurney C (2020) Out of harm's way? Critical remarks on harm and the meaning of home during the 2020 COVID-19 social distancing measures. Retrieved from https://housingevidence.ac.uk/publications/out-of-harms-way (accessed 22 July 2020).

Hine C (2020) Strategies for reflexive ethnography in the smart home: autoethnography of silence and emotion. *Sociology* 54 (1): 22–36.

Ingold T (2000) *The Perception of the Environment: Essays in Livelihood, Dwelling and Skill*. New York: Routledge.

Ingold T (2007) *Being Alive: Essays on Movement, Knowledge and Description*. New York: Routledge.

Martella F and Enia M (2020) Towards an urban domesticity. Contemporary architecture and the blurring boundaries between the house and the city. *Housing, Theory and Society* 37 (4): 1–17.

Mol A 2002*The Body Multiple: Ontology in Medical Practice*. Durham, NC: Duke University Press.

Otte J (2020) 'Everything will be all right': message of hope spreads in Italy. *The Guardian*, 12 March. Retrieved from www.theguardian.com/world/2020/mar/12/everything-will-be-a lright-italians-share-slogan-of-hope-in-face-of-coronavirus-crisis (accessed 25 August 2020).
Perec G (1997) *Species of Spaces and Other Pieces*. London: Penguin Books.
Rabinow P (2009) *Anthropos Today: Reflections on Modern Equipment*. Princeton, NJ: Princeton University Press.
Roy M, Moreau N, Rousseau C, Mercier A, Wilson A and Atlani-Duault L (2020) Ebola and localized blame on social media: analysis of Twitter and Facebook conversations during the 2014–2015 Ebola epidemic. *Culture, Medicine, and Psychiatry* 44 (1): 56–79.
Scambler G (2020) Covid-19 as a 'breaching experiment': exposing the fractured society. *Health Sociology Review* 29 (2): 1–9.
Soaita AM and McKee K (2019) Assembling a 'kind of' home in the UK private renting sector. *Geoforum* 103, July: 148–157.
Sundell Jet al. (2011) Ventilation rates and health: multidisciplinary review of the scientific literature. *Indoor Air* 21 (3): 191–204.
Van Loon J (2005) Epidemic space. *Critical Public Health* 15 (1): 39–52.
Whatmore S (2006) Materialist returns: practising cultural geography in and for a more-than-human world. *Cultural Geographies* 13 (4): 600–609.

6

THE POLITICS OF TOUCH-BASED HELP FOR VISUALLY IMPAIRED PERSONS DURING THE COVID-19 PANDEMIC

An autoethnographic account

Heidi Lourens

In memory of Heidi Volkwijn

Introduction

It is a chilly winter's morning in South Africa. Fearing the cold that surely awaits outside, I linger a bit longer under the cosiness of my duvet. Trying not to disturb my cat, which is curled up on my chest, I stretch out my arm to grab my phone on the bedside table. Let's see what's happening on Facebook, I lazily think to myself. Mmm, it's someone's birthday – got to remember to wish her many happy returns. I chuckle as I read another friend's comical update on the adventures of her cats. And then, without warning, I read it – an informal tribute to Heidi Volkwijn. The shock is visceral. I am shaking uncontrollably. The coronavirus took someone's life – someone who I've met before, someone whose hand I shook three years ago, someone who sat next to me in a meeting, someone whose perfume I smelled. The coronavirus took someone's life – someone, who, like me, is blind, someone who shares my name and someone, who, like me, is younger than 45 years old.

Barely three months ago, a local radio host conducted an interview with Heidi Volkwijn to discuss the particular vulnerabilities of people with visual impairments during the time of the COVID-19 pandemic. I clearly remember her words:

> Being blind or visually impaired, one's sense of touch is a very important sense, because this is how somebody who is blind or visually impaired gets to explore the world around them, gets to experience their environment. And with this virus, it of course impacts your ability, because now everything is heightened. You know, in terms of, I need to limit what I'm touching, I need to limit the physical contact that I'm making with surfaces, with areas, with people.
>
> *(Radio 702, 2020)*

Whether Heidi died because of her particular disability-related vulnerabilities I do not know. What I do know is that she is blind and that she passed away after becoming ill with COVID.

Of course, thousands of people die from COVID on a daily basis – people from all races, religions and abilities. But Heidi died and she was blind. And this fact slams it home for me and heightens my anxieties.

In this chapter, I will use the method of evocative autoethnography to discuss the myriad psychological and relational dimensions of help for visually impaired persons in the time of COVID. I will argue that, because help for people living with such impairments is often synonymous with touch (Goggin and Ellis, 2020; Health-e, 2020), it takes on different complexities within this time of social distancing and lockdown. These complexities rob me of minor freedoms – freedoms that are afforded to sighted persons even during regulated restrictions on movement. I conclude this essay with practical and theoretical perspectives on how to navigate this uncharted territory. But first, it is important to outline the complexities involved in the 'normal' day-to-day helping dynamics between disabled and nondisabled people. For even in pandemic-free times, the provision of help carries within it the potential for troublesome and 'sticky' relational and psychological dimensions (Lourens, 2018; Lourens et al., 2019; Watermeyer and Swartz, 2008).

Disability and the psychological dimensions of help

I have just arrived home from work. As is my custom, I first walk to the kettle to make myself a well-deserved cup of coffee. I pour the coffee grains, the sugar and wait for the kettle to boil. As I open the fridge, I realise, with a sinking feeling, that I forgot to buy milk. I really am not in the mood for black coffee, so I call my guide dog. 'Come boy, we're not yet done working.' I sigh while I grab my handbag, put the harness on my guide dog and open the front door. This is not going to be fun. It's peak traffic time. My dog wags his tail and pants while I lock my gate. His elation just serves to highlight my own irritation. As we approach the intersection, I suddenly feel a hand on my arm, pulling me towards the street. I jump. 'Wow, you frightened me,' I laugh. No reply. 'Hi, I'm Heidi.' I try to be polite. No reply. Finally, we cross the street and the stranger lets go of my arm. 'Thanks,' I mutter, not really succeeding in hiding my disgruntlement.

As I walked away from the 'helpful' stranger, I experienced a whole mix of emotions. I felt angry that he/she did not bother to greet me or ask whether I needed help. I felt worthless, because, surely, I thought, if someone could simply grab my arm without my permission, they think of me in some way as 'lesser than' themselves. And, probably heaviest of all the emotions, I felt guilty for feeling angry and irritated. The stranger was just trying to help, I sternly reprimanded myself. I also felt unable to voice my disgruntlement and frustration, because how do you tell someone who is 'just trying to help' that you don't want their help? How am I supposed to say something like that without appearing rude and ungrateful?

These feelings are not at all unfamiliar to me. For me, receiving help is often muddled with conflicting and uncomfortable emotions. And in this I am not alone. Many scholars have argued that in the context of disability, where the need for others' assistance is often assumed, such assistance might leave the help-recipients feeling dependent, worthless and disempowered (Lourens et al., 2019; Mik-Meyer, 2016; Shakespeare, 2000). I am not arguing here that the provision of help does not come with the best of intentions – it often does – but the execution of it often fails to consider the actual needs of the disabled person (Lourens et al., 2019). In the encounter sketched above, it would seem like there was no question in the stranger's mind that I definitely needed help. If there was any doubt in his/her mind, I assume that he/she would have asked me whether I needed assistance. But, because of the stereotypical assumption that disabled persons, by default, require help, I was the recipient of deeply unhelpful and unsolicited assistance.

In making this argument, I do not wish to suggest that I never welcome or need help. Of course I do. In fact, more often than not, I appreciate an offer of help to cross the street. But what I'm arguing here is that, ironically, my needs were not considered in the example sketched above. It felt like I was not approached as a 'whole' human being, but rather as an object that 'obviously' needed assistance. In this encounter, I was not afforded the opportunity to agree or refuse help because the stranger was not interested in my voice.

What may, in some instances, spark this non-conceptual provision of help, is the 'psychic pay-off' it may provide to help-providers (Marks, 1999). In helping non-disabled people, providers may gain a sense that they have contributed in a positive way to someone else's well-being. In this way, help may supply them with a sense of control and affirm their positive self-identity (Lourens et al., 2019; Marks, 1999). Seen from the opposite perspective, there are another set of feelings that the request for help might evoke for help-providers. In instances where disabled persons ask for help, nondisabled help-providers (albeit friends, strangers, colleagues and so on) might feel like they have no choice but to provide help (Lourens et al., 2019; Watermeyer and Swartz, 2008). Take, for example, a scenario in which I ask a friend to take me to the doctor. Of course, objectively speaking, my friend does have the right to refuse to help me in this regard. The point here is whether he would feel like he has the 'luxury' to say no and whether he would feel compelled by some form of moral duty to agree to something for which I clearly need help. Watermeyer and Swartz (2008: 606) aptly observe that, for nondisabled help-providers, there might exist the fantasy that 'I don't believe that you can cope with me being honest or with me not doing what you need me to do'.

It is thus clear that help, in the context of disability, is often drenched with numerous silences (Lourens, 2018; Lourens et al., 2019). Disabled people are often silent about their actual needs in helping encounters and relationships. And, like myself, some disabled people might hide their resentment and anger when on the receiving end of unsolicited help (Lourens et al., 2019). On the opposite end, help-providers may feel forced to provide help to disabled people – leaving them voiceless in their freedom to choose whether, indeed, they are willing or able to provide the requested help (Watermeyer and Swartz, 2008). And so, in these silent spaces between help-provider and help-recipient, the freedom of authentic communication is lost (Lourens et al., 2019). In these informal and formal helping relationships, it becomes more important to keep things polite and friendly, rather than paying the imagined price of voicing real feelings (Shakespeare, 2000).

The receipt and provision of help, in the context of disability, is thus anything but straightforward. Instead, it is intertwined with psychological complexities and entanglements. What I wanted to show in this section was that, even in the absence of the COVID pandemic, help already contained the potential for troublesome and 'sticky' relational and psychological dimensions (Lourens, 2018; Lourens et al., 2019; Watermeyer and Swartz, 2008). But in the current time of the pandemic, there is an added dimension to assistance when it applies to visually impaired persons. Here I am referring to the current dangers inherent to touch and the ways in which it further muddles formal and informal helping relationships for visually impaired people and their help-providers.

The coronavirus, visual impairment and the politics of touch-based help

Medical professionals mostly agree that viral respiratory infections, such as the current novel coronavirus, could be transmitted through direct contact with infected people, among other routes (Morawska and Cao, 2020). When infected people, for example, cough or sneeze on their hands and go on to touch an uninfected individual, the latter is directly exposed to infection. Yet, direct contact through physical touch is not the only means of contracting respiratory infections such as the novel coronavirus. Coming in close proximity to someone who has contracted the virus also would put someone at risk, because of airborne droplets that are released when the infected person sneezes or coughs (Morawska and Cao, 2020). Given all these risk factors, the World Health Organization (2020) recommends wearing a face mask in public, frequent hand sanitising and keeping a physical distance (at least one metre) from each other. It is therefore safe to say that, in this time of the coronavirus pandemic, touch has become synonymous with danger and threat, while those who choose to ignore the rules of social distancing and hygiene are often perceived to be irresponsible and selfish.

Yet, even in this time where touch has become a definite taboo, visually impaired people cannot divorce themselves from touch – it is an integral part of how they conduct their daily lives and move around in space (Giudice, 2020; Goggin and Ellis, 2020). As a visually impaired person, I frequently touch door-knobs, railings, arms of sighted guides, and so the list goes on. If I cannot touch my surroundings, I feel extremely disorientated and anxious – like I have been robbed of yet another sense. As another visually impaired person writes, 'The loss of these small but significant forms of contact because of pandemic-related concerns often leaves me feeling adrift, unfocused, and less connected to those around me' (Giudice, 2020). I imagine the unsettlement that Giudice describes here would be akin to requesting a sighted person to wear a blindfold in public. It is, to say the least, deeply distressing.

But, as distressing as the current demonisation of touch is for me, my association with touch has become equally anxiety-provoking. And so I am caught between a rock and a hard place. I desperately need to rely on touch in order to receive help, but I fear its potentially fatal consequences. Since the outbreak of the coronavirus, touch-based help contains more than the psychological and relational dimensions sketched thus far. Touch now contains an added dimension – it is now also intertwined with physical vulnerability and danger (Dickinson et al., 2020; Jalali et al., 2020).

In the previous section I have outlined the emotional responses that unsolicited help and touch evoke for me. While I always feel that such assistance is disrespectful and intrusive, I am now downright terrified of it. And, unfortunately, it continues despite the global push for social distancing. Recently, for example, my husband and I went to the supermarket. While I waited for my husband to choose our preferred washing powder, a woman walked up to me.

'Lovely dog,' she remarked, and simultaneously bent down to pat my guide dog.

'He is lovely, isn't he?' I smiled, even though I felt that she violated the rules of physical distancing. 'Well, you look after mommy,' she cooed and started to sympathetically rub my arm.

My entire body stiffened. In this encounter, I felt extremely vulnerable. Not only was I not consulted as to whether she could rub my arm, but in the process she potentially placed us both in danger. This left me wondering whether she thought, as others might, that disabled people cannot contract something deadly like the coronavirus. Some of my blind friends relayed similar experiences to me in many conversations that followed this encounter.

But then, as stated before, there are instances where I do need help and, in order to receive help, I do need to touch my help-provider. I cannot, for example, locate groceries in a supermarket without the help of a sighted person. In a BBC (2020) article, a visually impaired customer recalled his visit to a supermarket:

> They said they were not sure they could help because of 'current things going on,' he says. I guess it was a contact thing, because of having to take someone's arm for guiding. I waited around for over five minutes, and in the end they did help.

Currently, my reliance on touch-based help leaves me ashamed and guilt-ridden. As Giudice writes, 'I feel shamed by my affiliation with touch and my need to rely on this modality' (Giudice, 2020). In order to alleviate some of these shameful feelings, I sanitise my hands in front of the shop assistant, to show her that I take responsibility to protect her safety. But is it enough? As outlined in the previous section, sighted persons sometimes do feel obligated to provide help to disabled persons (Lourens et al., 2019). While walking with shop assistants, I do wonder whether they feel comfortable to be in close proximity to me. And, if not, do they feel comfortable expressing their discomfort?

And so, initially, when social distancing came into effect in South Africa, the shop assistant and I wove our way through the aisles of the supermarket, not uttering a word about the situation we were clearly locked into. We walked, located groceries and chatted about mundane matters of the day, not knowing what the other person thought, not knowing what the other person felt behind the masks we were wearing. I always felt guilt and shame – but what she felt I did not know.

So, after a few visits to the supermarket, I started leaving the shopping duties to my husband. In order to avoid the guilt, the shame and the 'not knowing what the shop assistant felt', I stayed at home – even after lockdown was lifted in our area. Most people would probably agree that was the sensible, responsible and less selfish choice. Yet, never leaving my home, never feeling the wondrous feeling of independence while I jog with my guide dog down the street, took an intense emotional toll on me. It is not uncommon for people to experience high levels of anxiety and depression during this time of confinement and social distancing (Brooks et al., 2020; Zhou et al., 2020). In a short space of time, my world shrank to the confined bars of my homely prison cell.

I know that all of us need to make sacrifices that sometimes feel unbearable: all of us have a moral duty to protect each other against the coronavirus. I therefore don't suggest, for one moment, that we throw caution to the wind and follow our 'hearts' in venturing outside. But I believe that the relational ethics of care can offer some guidelines for the ways in which visually impaired persons can navigate the outside world during the time of the COVID pandemic. While it is probable that most encounters with shop assistants will be brief and fleeting and thus not really relational, I want to argue here that even in the absence of relationship, even in the briefest of encounters, we can apply a relational ethics of care approach. These principles, I believe, can be applied from moment to moment with strangers who intersect our paths.

Arguing for a relational ethics of care during the COVID pandemic

It has been almost two weeks since the first coronavirus case was announced in South Africa. Ever since that day, I have managed to avoid the supermarket. But now, my husband has flu and it is up to me to buy some necessities for our home. As I cross the street to the supermarket, I experience an overwhelming sense of trepidation. Would the shop assistant be able to help me during this time of social distancing? Would she feel 'free' to voice her concerns if she experienced any? Would I put her or myself in danger?

As I stand in the doorway of the supermarket, I hear a familiar voice, 'Hello, Heidi. How are you?' 'I'm fine,' I greet the shop assistant who regularly helps me in the store. 'What are you buying today?' she says as she grabs a shopping basket. 'Just hold on,' I say while I take my hand sanitiser from my bag and spray it on my hands. She chuckles. 'Me too,' she says, while holding out her hands.

It was as if, in this mutual recognition of our vulnerability and shared responsibility to one another, we couldn't help but burst out laughing. Of course, there was really nothing funny about this encounter – it was an overt recognition of our frailty during this pandemic-ridden time – but, I think our laughter signified in some way that 'wow, we are together in these muddied waters'. And in this real and genuine exchange, I felt truly engaged and connected to this help-provider in our shared vulnerability and our mutual 'not knowing'. It felt like I was saying, 'I take responsibility to not infect you.' And she was reciprocating the same message to me. In this encounter, we showed 'mutual respect' for each other: a cornerstone of the relational ethics of care (Bergum and Dossetor, 2005; Cloutier et al., 2015). Here I do not refer to care in its traditional virtuous sense – I refer to it as a practice that serves to improve the well-being of another (Branicki, 2020; Noddings, 2003). In this sense, the shop assistant and I showed care for one another, as silently and respectfully we acknowledged that 'what I do affects you, and what you do affects me' (Bergum and Dossetor, 2005).

While mutual respect is crucial during these times, I believe that another principle of the relational ethics of care is required to aid in the interaction between help-provider and help-recipient. What I am referring to here is the principle of engagement (Cloutier et al., 2015). First, engagement asks of us to see and recognise people – particularly those we help – as whole persons (Cloutier et al., 2015). To engage, in essence, means to 'reach a shared sense of the experience and of each other' (Way and Tracy 2012: 304). When the other is seen as a whole person, then 'the shift is from solving the ethical problem to asking the ethical question' (Bergum and Dossetor, 2005: 3).

In this time of pandemic – as always – it is important to open things up. In our interactions with each other, it becomes crucial to refrain from shying away from ethical dilemmas that threaten to shut us up. Earlier in this essay, I mentioned that in one of my initial encounters with a shop assistant at a supermarket, I felt uncomfortable in my guilt and shame. Similarly, I felt uncomfortable in the knowledge that I was not aware how the assistant felt helping me in a time when social closeness is an absolute taboo. But we both didn't utter a word about our feelings – we walked as if COVID was not the looming presence between us.

Recently, I deliberately decided to 'ask the ethical question'. I realised that if I wanted the freedom to move around independently, it would require something ethical from me. So now, if I visit the supermarket, I ask the shop assistant, 'Do you feel comfortable helping me?' and 'How do you prefer to help me?' I deliberately state that I don't want to put her in danger, so I also provide some practical options. 'If you guide me, I can take your shoulder. Or I can tell you what I want and you can go and get it while I wait for you?' Thus far, I have been fortunate enough that shop assistants were always willing to help me. This might not be the case for others and I'm not suggesting for one minute that this is a fool-proof solution. After all:

> Relational ethics of care are ongoing, uncertain processes. Often what is ethical to do in any situation may not be clear, but something must be done and/or decided. One is never finished making ethical decisions as long as [*sic*] interacting with others. Thus we must be fully present and continually asking questions about

> 'what is going on here,' in particular 'what is needed to make this interaction go well, to honor the other person, and to take care of myself?'.
>
> *(Ellis, 2016: 139)*

Of course, it could be argued that it is not fair for disabled persons to ask the ethical question and be burdened by the responsibility of navigating this ethical space. I agree. But in a time where decisions must be made quickly, I can only hope that my behaviour models something of the relational ethics of care to someone else. I am also not suggesting that the relational ethics of care is a fool-proof solution for the dilemmas sketched thus far. In an ideal world, I would want to see protocols that would guide help-providers and help-recipients in best practices to ensure their safety (Dickinson et al., 2020). But, in the absence of such protocols, I think it could help to start with open responsiveness to one another in our mutual recognition of each other's personhood.

Conclusion

In this essay I have outlined various psychological and relational entanglements of help in the context of disability. I have demonstrated the ways in which help is often infused with myriad silences where help-providers and help-recipients sometimes feel prohibited from voicing their real feelings and concerns regarding the help relationship. Following the outbreak of the COVID pandemic, these psychological and relational entanglements did not go away. To the contrary. Help, in the context of visual impairment, now has the added dimension of associations with touch. In turn, touch is one of the primary ways of contracting the deadly coronavirus. In light of this, an already complex phenomenon of help and disability becomes compounded by the fear of contracting the coronavirus. Intermingled with already complex helping encounters, there is also a mixture of guilt, shame and anxieties that are specific to associations with touch.

During this health crisis, it is important to revisit and reapply an ethics of care approach. What we need is to be open and reflexive in our responses to one another. Through open responsiveness to one another, disabled and nondisabled persons will come to learn what the unique realities and needs of each unique individual are (Kittay, 2006). In other words, only through authentic communication and active engagement will disabled and nondisabled persons recognise the unique context, needs and emotions of one another.

References

BBC (2020) Being blind during the pandemic. Retrieved from www.bbc.com/news/disability-52118942 (accessed 4 June 2020).

Bergum V and Dossetor J (2005) *Relational Ethics: The Full Meaning of Respect*. Hagerstown, MD: University Publishing Group.

Branicki LJ (2020) COVID-19, ethics of care and feminist crisis management. *Gender, Work & Organization* 27 (5): 872–883.

Brooks SK, Webster RK, Smith LEet al. (2020) The psychological impact of quarantine and how to reduce it: rapid review of the evidence. *Rapid Review* 395 (10227): 912–920.

Cloutier D, Martin-Matthews A, Byrne Ket al. (2015) The space between: using 'relational ethics' and 'relational space' to explore relationship-building between care providers and care recipients in the home space. *Social & Cultural Geography* 16 (7): 764–782.

Dickinson H, Carey G and Kavanagh AM (2020) Personalisation and pandemic: an unforeseen collision course? *Disability & Society* 35 (6): 1012–1017.

Ellis C (2016) Compassionate research: interviewing and storytelling from a relational ethics of care. In: Goodson I, Antikainen A, Sikes P and Andrews M (eds) *The Routledge International Handbook on Narrative and Life History*. London: Routledge, pp. 431–445.

Giudice NA (2020) COVID-19 and blindness: why the new touchless, physically-distant world sucks for people with visual impairment. Retrieved from https://medium.com/@nicholas.giudice/covid-19-and-blindness-why-the-new-touchless-physically-distant-world-sucks-for-people-with-2c8dbd21de63 (accessed 5 June 2020).

Goggin G and Ellis K (2020) Disability, communication, and life itself in the COVID-19 pandemic. *Health Sociology Review* 29 (2): 168–176.

Health-e (2020) Covid-19 makes life 'extra difficult' for the blind. Retrieved from https://health-e.org.za/2020/06/11/covid-19-makes-life-extra-difficult-for-the-blind (accessed 29 June 2020).

Jalali M, Shahabi S, Lankarani KBet al. (2020) COVID-19 and disabled people: perspectives from Iran. *Disability & Society* 35 (5): 844–847.

Kittay EF (2006) The concept of care ethics in biomedicine: the case of disability. In: Rehmann-Sutter C, Düwell M and Mieth D (eds) *Bioethics in Cultural Contexts*. Dordrecht: Springer, pp. 319–338.

Lourens H (2018) Driving in unheard silence: disability and the politics of shutting up. *Journal of Health Psychology* 23 (4): 567–576.

Lourens H, Watermeyer B and Swartz L (2019) Ties that bind, and double-bind: visual impairment, help, and the shaping of relationship. *Disability & Rehabilitation* 41 (16): 1890–1897.

Marks D (1999) Dimensions of oppression: theorising the embodied subject. *Disability & Society* 14 (5): 611–626.

Mik-Meyer N (2016) Disability and 'care': managers, employees and colleagues with impairments negotiating the social order of disability. *Work, Employment & Society* 30 (6): 984–999.

Morawska L and Cao G (2020) Airborne transmission of SARS-COV-2: the world should face the reality. *Environment International* 139. Retrieved from https://www.sciencedirect.com/science/article/pii/S016041202031254X?via%3Dihub (accessed 11 January 2021).

Noddings N (2003) *Caring: A Feminine Approach to Ethics and Moral Education* (2nd edition). Berkeley, CA: University of California Press.

Radio 702 (2020) Visually impaired people and Coronavirus. Retrieved from www.702.co.za/podcasts/269/tonight-with-lester-kiewit/298807/visually-impaired-people-and-coronavirus (accessed 15 June 2020).

Shakespeare T (2000) *Help*. Birmingham: Venture Press.

Watermeyer B and Swartz L (2008) Conceptualising the psycho-emotional aspects of disability and impairment: The distortion of personal and psychic boundaries. *Disability & Society* 23 (6): 599–610.

Way D and Tracy S (2012) Conceptualizing compassion as recognizing, relating and (re) acting: a qualitative study of compassionate communication at hospice. *Communication Monographs* 79 (3): 292–315.

World Health Organization (2020) Coronavirus disease (COVID-19) advice for the public. Retrieved from www.who.int/emergencies/diseases/novel-coronavirus-2019/advice-for-public (accessed 29 June 2020).

Zhou X, Snoswell CL, Harding LE et al. (2020) The role of telehealth in reducing the mental health burden from COVID-19. *Telemedicine and E-Health* 26 (4). Retrieved from https://www.liebertpub.com/doi/10.1089/tmj.2020.0068 (accessed 11 January 2021).

PART III

Intimacies, socialities and connections

7

#DATINGWHILEDISTANCING

Dating apps as digital health technologies during the COVID-19 pandemic

David Myles, Stefanie Duguay and Christopher Dietzel

Introduction

The COVID-19 pandemic has required governments and public health agencies to implement unprecedented physical and social distancing measures. By 2 April 2020, it was estimated that close to 4 billion individuals had been confined to their homes worldwide (Fahey, 2020). These measures have placed significant economic pressure on the service industries. This is also true for online dating services, and particularly for dating app companies that consider geographic proximity and mobility as key commodities. Initial contact between dating app users typically occurs online, but the promise of physical contact, whether romantic or sexual, is an important selling point used by these apps to market the services they offer. If dating apps experienced a rise in downloads at the start of the pandemic (Lehmiller et al., 2020; Petrychyn, 2020), physical distancing measures may ultimately decrease the value of digitally mediated dating services by making it more difficult for them to retain users, generate profit and remain culturally relevant. The COVID pandemic has also raised important issues surrounding the social responsibility that dating apps share in mitigating the spread of the novel coronavirus and, more generally, in protecting the health of their users.

This chapter examines how international dating app companies responded in the early months of the pandemic. Our preliminary findings suggest that these companies and their products emerged as important social actors who increasingly engaged in digital health using three strategies. First, they communicated health information to their user base and promoted dating habits that are in line with public health guidelines. Second, they play an active role in making physical distancing measures socially meaningful. Third, they enforce strategies to normalise dating practices that take place exclusively online, which can affect sexual and public health by reshaping contemporary dating cultures.

Dating apps and digital health

Dating apps were popularised in the early 2010s and result from the digitisation of dating services that began in the 1990s. These apps were first developed by, and catered to, queer men (with apps like Grindr and Scruff) before reaching heterosexual markets (with apps like Tinder and Bumble). Drawing on recent developments in smart telephony, dating apps provide new features to users, such as mobility and geolocation, and monetise their services by offering premium memberships, developing targeted advertisements and brokering user data. The services offered by dating apps are reshaping contemporary dating cultures in ways that generate important cultural (Duguay et al., 2017), commercial (Wilken et al., 2019) and sociotechnical implications (Licoppe et al., 2016), which have been raised by researchers in a variety of fields, including media and communication, sociology, cultural studies, and sexuality and gender studies.

Dating apps are also associated with important health-related issues (Albury et al., 2019). As such, they can be (and have been) understood as digital health technologies, even if their main objectives are not specifically health-related. By digital health technologies, we mean that dating apps are part of 'a wide range of technologies' that generally 'engage in activities to promote [individuals'] health and well-being and avoid illness' (Lupton, 2017: 1). Today, digital health technologies extend well beyond the strictly clinical or medical realm. Likewise, the researchers who engage with these technologies are increasingly moving beyond instrumental perspectives to examine them critically (Lupton, 2014). Over the past decade, researchers and health practitioners have identified the relations between dating apps and digital health in various ways. We detail three modes in this section: dating apps as health risk factors, dating apps as intervention tools, and dating apps as influential health actors.

After their initial entry into the dating space, dating apps were rapidly targeted by public health actors as potential *risk factors* for public and individual health, and especially for sexual health and wellbeing. Studies sought to explore the causality between the use of dating apps, on the one hand, and the increase in promiscuity and sexually transmitted infections (STIs) on the other (Shapiro et al., 2017). Researchers have particularly hypothesised the responsibility of dating apps in the spread of STIs among queer men (Mowlabocus et al., 2016). This is not surprising, as dating apps were first developed for and by queer men, whose sexual practices have been the target of continuing monitoring by public health authorities. Some studies considering dating apps as risk factors have been criticised for their tendency to reproduce techno-deterministic, and even technophobic, assumptions about the digital mediation of queer sexuality (Race, 2015). Nevertheless, these studies remain significant because they actively participated in grounding dating apps within the realm of digital health very early on.

Health researchers and practitioners have quickly identified dating apps as potential *tools* that could be leveraged to reach target populations. This perspective relies on the assumption that dating apps constitute sites that need to be invested in to perform digital health (Holloway et al., 2014). For example, studies have mobilised apps to promote 'healthy' dating or hook-up practices (Thompson et al., 2019), help monitor STI outbreaks and spread (Beebeejaun et al., 2017) and conduct recruitment for population surveys (Goedel & Duncan, 2015). In these studies, dating apps are generally understood as being the hosts for external digital health initiatives that seek to document and eventually change dating or hook-up habits among users.

Today, dating apps are taking on increasingly active roles as social *actors* who implicate themselves in digital health. Dating app companies – especially those catering to queer men – have enforced their own initiatives to promote 'safe' dating habits and to reduce risks related to health and safety. For example, Grindr has recently 'healthicised' – to borrow from Conrad (1992) – part of its services to queer users by introducing profile categories that relate to serological status and STI screening habits. Dating app companies also develop partnerships with third-party collaborators to sell pharmaceutical products or provide medical services and appointments to their users, among other initiatives. In these cases, dating apps internally engage in digital health as responsive actors and not simply as tools invested in, or used by, external health actors.

Our study: monitoring dating app responses during the pandemic

The COVID pandemic is a uniquely rich case study for examining the role of dating apps as responsive to digital health. To document the initial responses of dating apps in the context of increased governmental and economic pressure, we engaged in a study building on the app walkthrough method, which generally seeks to provide a 'detailed analysis of an app's intended purpose, embedded cultural meanings and implied ideal users and uses' (Light et al., 2018: 881).

In this chapter, we draw on data collected over three months (March to May 2020) and three types of terrain. First, to document how dating apps communicated directly with their users and adapted their services, we conducted non-participant observation on 16 dating apps (Ashley Madison, Bumble, Coffee Meets Bagel, Grindr, Growlr, Happn, Her, Hinge, Hornet, Jack'd, Lex, Match, OkCupid, Plenty of Fish, Scruff, Tinder). We signed up as users and gradually collected screenshots of relevant material. Second, we collected COVID-related posts produced by these dating app companies on their Instagram accounts, corporate blogs and websites. Through these first two steps, we collected 2298 app screenshots, 97 blog posts and 10 press releases that were the objects of our analysis. Third, we collected 188 newspaper and magazine articles (published in English, mostly from American, Australian, British, Canadian, and New Zealand sources) via the Google News search engine (by searching keywords like dating app, pandemic, COVID-19, Tinder, Grindr etc.) to monitor the public discourses and controversies relating to online dating in the time of the COVID, which we used to contextualise our initial findings. The following sections present the preliminary results of our analysis.

Communicating health guidelines

Like many popular social media platforms, dating app companies started communicating with their users about the risks related to the novel coronavirus by mid-March 2020. They first did so by using in-app communication features like pop-up messages. These pop-ups were used to highlight the individual responsibility of each user to practise physical distancing. Users were quickly asked to stop meeting in-person and limit their dating or sexual activities to online interactions. Dating apps particularly used pop-up features to mobilise their publics by speaking to a sense of belonging and community. For example, Tinder wrote to its users: 'Keeping yourself safe and healthy helps to keep everyone in our community safe and healthy, too'. The company added: 'Social distancing doesn't have to mean disconnecting'. Similarly, Scruff sent this message: 'Remember that being physically distanced from each other does not mean we're alone'. Grindr summarised the situation as: 'Isolated but not alone'. Dating app companies also sought to reduce collective fears by emphasising that everything was going to be all right.

Overall, in-app communications allowed dating app companies to reinterpret their mission statement in light of the COVID pandemic, which was now to leverage their services to alleviate their users' loneliness, facilitate their confinement and potentially prevent new transmissions. In the following weeks, in-app features were increasingly used to perform health promotion and share official public health guidelines. Users were invited to stay home, wash their hands, practise physical distancing and consult a doctor if they experienced fever or respiratory difficulties, among other recommendations. Dating apps also acted as public health intermediaries by redirecting their users to external public health resources from local (provincial or state agencies), national (Centers for Disease Control and Prevention, Health Canada) and transnational (World Health Organization) sources.

Dating apps that cater to queer men were particularly active in health communication. For example, Hornet quickly reminded its user base about the importance of stocking HIV medicine. It also mobilised health ambassadors (typically used for STI- and HIV-related social support) to answer COVID-related questions locally, thus re-distributing digital health labour within the community. Grindr shared mental, sexual and physical health resources that were adapted to its publics. In Canada, the app shared links to CATIE, a source of HIV/hepatitis C information, and Prepster, a UK-based information source on HIV treatment, to provide users with information on the risks that the novel coronavirus presented for immunosuppressed people. Interestingly, it also used a pre-existing HIV monitoring strategy to help track down individuals potentially infected by the coronavirus. Users who received a positive SARS-CoV-2 result were invited to contact Grindr with the identities of their latest partners, who would then be notified anonymously. In these ways, apps that cater to queer men engaged more quickly and actively in digital health labour, arguably because of their previous experience in monitoring viral transmissions within their user base.

In-app communications were not exclusively used to engage in digital health but were also mobilised in marketing ploys. Several dating apps used pop-ups to publicise their community events such as music concerts, Q&As and dating advice sessions. Some apps shared health-related advertisements to further commodify their user base during the COVID pandemic. For example, Scruff offered free soap products with the purchase of affiliate merchandise, while Grindr promoted N-95 masks that could 'save your life'. To do so, Grindr shared on Instagram the catchphrase 'mask for mask', a play on words that draws on gay cruising cultures where masculine (or 'masc') men are often considered more desirable. Furthermore, several dating apps created or unlocked exclusive features for a limited time to increase user engagement. These features were most commonly labelled as 'gifts' or 'rewards' and marketed to users as a way to ease their confinement. For example, several apps (like Bumble, Grindr, Hinge, Jack'd, Match and Plenty of Fish) offered members free video services, Scruff increased the number of accessible grid profiles and Lex raised the number of daily posts allowed. Tinder remarketed its passport feature to facilitate transnational matching, a feature relying heavily on the metaphor of travel that sought to recreate the experience of mobility.

While these features were presented as gifts to reward users for staying home, they also enacted a marketing strategy to retain users and potentially increase the number of premium subscriptions upon making these features exclusive again. Thus, as dating apps rapidly took on the role of digital health intermediaries, their communications intersected, and often blurred, public health and commercial imperatives.

Making distancing measures socially meaningful

The contribution of dating app companies to digital health is not limited to communicating risks and public health guidelines. These companies also attempted to make physical distancing measures meaningful and socially acceptable, especially through their social media accounts and blogging platforms. The COVID pandemic and the numerous calls for physical distancing presented significant challenges for the business model of dating app companies. Going on a 'virtual date' might appear frivolous for some in the context of a major global crisis, and prospective users might ask themselves what is the point of dating, given the restrictions on in-person encounters and physical contact. Inversely, the pandemic also presented the opportunity for dating app companies to change people's perceptions of what online dating means and has to offer by illustrating how it could facilitate physical distancing. Our initial observations suggest that as dating app companies attempted to reinforce the social acceptance of physical distancing measures, they often did so for their own benefit by strategically conflating the merits of physical distancing and online dating. In turn, conflating 'staying at home' and 'dating while distancing' allowed for dating app companies to subvert some of the ongoing criticisms they have received over the past decade.

One of the main benefits of online dating in the context of the COVID pandemic is that, as opposed to in-person encounters, virtual dates cannot result in viral transmissions. Thus, dating from the comfort of one's home was portrayed as a safer option. The idea that online dating is 'safe' subverts a decade of criticisms that underscore the alleged perils of dating apps. These apps have persistently been accused of encouraging criminal behaviours (such as nefarious lurking, identity fraud and catfishing, physical and sexual assaults) (Kjellson, 2016) and harming the health and safety of their users (such as online harassment, self-esteem decline and STI transmission) (Gollom, 2016; Turban, 2018). While some of these reservations are founded, as shown by the negative experiences shared by many female, queer and/or racialised dating app users (Bivens & Hoque, 2018; Daroya, 2017), others are instead the result of technophobic and sex-negative moral panics (Ahlm, 2017). Nevertheless, the COVID pandemic enabled dating app companies to portray their apps as being the safest option right now, thus demonstrating how risk is always assessed and negotiated contextually. Online dating was not only depicted as being safer: since confinement measures can lead to social isolation, dating apps were also presented as beneficial tools that facilitate meaningful intimate connections, thereby supporting the mental and emotional health of single people, especially those who live alone.

To promote online dating as beneficial, companies mobilised discourses underlining the importance of self-care and personal wellbeing. Dating while distancing was portrayed as a proactive way of taking care of one's self and reducing loneliness through social interactions. Moreover, dating app companies countered the assumption that online dating consists of a somewhat frivolous activity in these serious times. On the contrary, staying home was likened to a social responsibility or even a civic duty that responds to public health and societal imperatives, thus making dating or flirting while distancing seem like a heroic or political act. This message is well illustrated by the queer app Lex, which shared user posts on Instagram encouraging others to send nudes to essential workers. One post read: 'Nudes 4 Essential Workers. You're on the frontlines and I love you for it. Let me distract & destress you with some flirty pics.' Other queer apps, like Grindr, Hornet and Scruff, also heavily relied on making isolation sexy by sharing erotic pictures of their users stuck at home yet making the best of their confinement. These apps eroticised bio-politicised subjects by promoting the belief that social distancing was a sexy or desirable quality. Overall, queer apps addressed sexuality and virtual hook-ups more explicitly and in a more sex-positive manner than their mainstream counterparts, often discussing sexting, pornography, synchronous video sex parties and other means of digitally-mediated sexual activities and expression.

In contrast, apps that cater to predominantly heterosexual publics (like Coffee Meets Bagel, Hinge, Match, OkCupid, Plenty of Fish and Tinder) promoted posts that shared a more romantic view of online dating. Physical distancing measures were shown as the opportunity for dating app users to plan imaginative video dates and foster 'real' connections that moved beyond instant sexual gratification. Overall, physical distancing measures allowed dating app companies to subvert the assumption that online dating is shameful or something to hide. One example of this messaging included a Tinder post to Instagram sharing a tweet from comedian

Dan LaMorte stating: 'Remember when everyone hid that they met online and now it's like, "Ew, you met in society?"' The circulation of such messages pushed back against taboos that still surround online dating today, regardless of its growing popularity (Khoury, 2018). The active search to meet partners online – as opposed to meeting partners physically – could now be portrayed as a desirable and even honourable action, one that newly formed couples might even shape into venerable stories to share with their future children.

Normalising online dating cultures

Dating app companies can also be understood as digital health actors because they normalise online dating cultures and practices in ways that can impact the physical, mental and sexual health of their users. These companies circulate the belief that it is socially acceptable for users to date online and standardise how it should occur by providing tips and guidance. Thus, they have become new moral authorities that participate in shaping attitudes and behaviours in matters of human sexuality, romance, flirting, partnering and socialisation. However, physical distancing measures required dating app companies to considerably adjust their usual dating advice, which has typically been geared towards facilitating quick and easy face-to-face meetups. To do so, dating apps subverted recurring tropes in online dating cultures on their social media accounts. On Instagram, Tinder posted the phrase '~~Not~~ looking for a penpal' to challenge the widespread belief that long, text-based conversations on dating apps are tedious and boring. Similarly, Grindr circulated the phrase '"Right Now" can wait' to subvert its usual emphasis on physical proximity and immediacy.

Our initial findings point to various strategies developed by dating apps to normalise online dating. Several apps, including Bumble, Coffee Meets Bagel, Hinge, Match, OkCupid, Plenty of Fish and Tinder, shared statistics that showed increasing interest in digitally-mediated dating services during the pandemic to reassure potential users that they were not alone in turning to apps or the internet to meet potential partners. These statistics might also have been shared to underline how dating apps remained socially relevant and financially viable, especially to investors. Moreover, OkCupid shared a series of catchphrases that further sought to normalise the prospect of online dating during the pandemic by using the template 'It's ok to …'. For example, OkCupid posted 'It's ok to walk 6 [feet] apart even if you believe size doesn't matter' and 'It's ok to love clean hands and dirty talk'. Many apps (like Match, which coined the hashtag #DatingWhileDistancing) curated memes and jokes about real-life situations that showed the banal yet strange and awkward occurrences that take place when dating from home, signalling to users that they were not alone in experiencing these events. In a way, these posts illustrated the new 'normal' of dating.

Dating app companies also actively engaged in providing their users with dating tips particularly geared at guiding them through 'virtual dates'. Most apps used their social media accounts, blogging platforms or pop-up features to provide users with a series of guides to help them adapt to, and perfect their behaviours for, video-based meetups. These guides addressed interpersonal communication skills, conversation topics, fashion advice and suggestions for date activities. Some apps also invited dating coaches to share their expertise during live video events. Unsurprisingly, the circulation of these guides and coaching sessions sometimes coincided with the promotion of (paid) app features and sponsored events specifically marketed to facilitate virtual dates. While these guides were portrayed as resources to help users interact online, they also constituted in-house advertisements that prompted customers into purchasing or maximising the use of specific app features. Thus, dating guides were also marketing ploys where new features were introduced and their benefits explained.

The COVID pandemic was particularly useful for apps to introduce and experiment with new video and audio features that prompted users to move beyond casual texting. Physical distancing measures meant that first dates would now have to occur online via video. While some apps like Tinder and Her invited their user base to explore external video services (like Zoom, Skype and FaceTime), others promoted their in-house video services, like Grindr, which offered two minutes of free video conversation every day, after which the feature became a paid service. The move from textual to video-based interactions also prompted apps to introduce features to manage consent and user insecurities, as video-based dates can be somewhat challenging. For example, Bumble introduced the 'virtual date badge' that users could place on their personal profile to help them find other people also interested in video chats. Similarly, Hinge introduced 'Date from Home', a double opt-in video feature that members could use to secretly communicate their willingness to move from texting to a virtual date when (and only if) both parties clicked on the feature. Thus, the COVID pandemic represented an experimental ground for dating app companies to facilitate dating while distancing, while also prompting them to manage the ambivalence and vulnerabilities of their user base by providing new features and prescribing appropriate dating etiquette to navigate these uncertain times.

Future provocations

This chapter has examined the discursive and technological strategies through which dating apps positioned themselves as unconventional corporate digital health technologies during the early stages of the COVID pandemic by circulating public health guidelines and shaping acceptable dating practices during times of physical distancing. It illustrates how dating app companies are subverting negative associations with online dating to incentivise the use of new features and approaches to dating 'virtually' without physical contact. This study points to new research directions as the pandemic unfolds and the responses of dating app companies continue to evolve.

Our preliminary observations suggest that dating app companies are leveraging physical distancing measures to reshape online dating as a collective endeavour rather than a strictly individual one. This is mainly attempted by speaking to their users' feeling of community, especially among apps whose mission statements already contain explicit sociopolitical goals. For example, Bumble, a self-proclaimed feminist app that mainly targets heterosexual women, shared political content to celebrate the work done by healthcare professionals who are mostly female. Apps like Her and Lex, both developed for queer women, organised multiple online community events, shared political statements on their social media accounts (for example, in relation to the 'Cancel rent' campaign) and instigated aid relief initiatives to support queer women and businesses that may be struggling financially. Calls for unity and community were also prominent in queer apps like Grindr and Scruff, especially to protect the most vulnerable members of the LGBTQ+ communities who may be street-involved, immunosuppressed, or in financially precarious situations.

'Community' is a polysemic term, and our initial observations suggest tensions and overlaps between communities of users (that is, the sum of individuals who use a single dating app) and pre-existing communities based on common sociodemographic characteristics (like sexual and gender categories). While calls to unity were also observed in more mainstream apps, what 'community' means in those contexts remains unclear. For example, when Tinder, a mainstream app that operates in over 200 countries, urges users to stay at home to protect the 'community', what does that entail? Does this refer to all Tinder users? To users that belong to local communities or geographically-bound territories? On the one hand, calls to community may be deployed to reassure users that there is still hope, that things will get better and that social institutions will endure this crisis. On the other hand, this trope might also be a marketing ploy used by dating app companies to make their services relevant and, therefore, valuable in the context of the COVID pandemic. As such, the various meanings and strategic use of the term 'community' (among other corporate metaphors like 'self-care', 'gift' or 'wellbeing') require further examination.

Beyond public relations and marketing campaigns, future research is needed to investigate the corporate practices that dating app companies implement and their consequences in light of the commercial imperatives under which they operate. These practices not only have an impact on sexual and public health; they raise social justice issues, especially in relation to the increasing trends in epidemiological research that rely on populational monitoring via digital media platforms. Future research that examines the responses of dating apps during future phases of the COVID crisis should address offstage corporate decisions that further expand the surveillance and tracking of users in ways that may challenge fundamental rights to privacy and self-determination.

Finally, future research could investigate the potential value of dating app data for epidemiological research. For example, what kinds of data publics are dating app services generating during the COVID pandemic? And what third parties are acquiring these datasets, for what purposes and under which regulatory bodies? Ultimately, when dating apps act as digital health actors in times of crisis, they should be comparably held to the standards under which operate the formal health institutions that affect, support or sustain public health. We point to these provocations for future research to highlight the need for serious scholarly consideration of dating apps as they shape the public health landscape through the normalisation, datafication and commodification of contemporary dating cultures.

References

Ahlm J (2017) Respectable promiscuity: digital cruising in an era of queer liberalism. *Sexualities* 20 (3): 364–379.

Albury K, Byron P, McCosker A, Pym T, Walshe J, Race K, Salon D, Wark T, Botfield J, Reeders D and Dietzel C (2019) *Safety, Risk and Wellbeing on Dating Apps*. Final report, December. Melbourne, Australia: Swinburne University of Technology.

Beebeejaun K, Degala S, Balogun K, Simms I, Woodhall SC, Heinsbroek E, Crook, PD, Kar-Purkayastha I, Treacy J, Wedgwood K, Jordan K, Mandal S, Ngui SL and Edelstein M (2017) Outbreak of hepatitis A associated with men who have sex with men (MSM), England, July 2016 to January 2017. *Eurosurveillance* 22 (5): 30454.

Bivens R and Hoque AS (2018). Programming sex, gender, and sexuality: infrastructural failures in the 'feminist' dating app Bumble. *Canadian Journal of Communication* 43 (3): 441–459.

Conrad P (1992) Medicalization and social control. *Annual Review of Sociology* 18 (1): 209–232.

Daroya E (2017) Erotic capital and the psychic life of racism on Grindr. In: Riggs DW (ed.) *The Psychic Life of Racism in Gay Men's Communities*. Lanham, MD: Lexington Books, pp. 67–80.

Duguay S, Burgess J and Light B (2017) Mobile dating and hookup app culture. In: Messaris P and Humphreys L (eds) *Digital Media: Transformations in Human Communication* (2nd edn). New York: Peter Lang, pp. 213–221.

Fahey R (2020) Half the world in lockdown. *Daily Mail*, April 2. Retrieved from www.dailymail.co.uk/news/article-8181001/3-9-billion-people-currently-called-stay-homes-coronavirus.html (accessed 2 April 2020).

Goedel WC and Duncan DT (2015) Geosocial-networking app usage patterns of gay, bisexual, and other men who have sex with men: survey among users of Grindr, a mobile dating app. *JMIR Public Health and Surveillance* 1 (1). Retrieved from https://publichealth.jmir.org/2015/1/e4/ (accessed 11 January 2021).

Gollom M (2016) Blame Tinder, Grindr for the rise in sexually transmitted diseases? Not so fast. *CBC News*, 29 April. Retrieved from www.cbc.ca/news/health/tinder-grindr-alberta-sti-outbreak-1.3555639 (accessed 29 March 2019).

Holloway IW, Rice E, Gibbs J, Winetrobe H, Dunlap S and Rhoades H (2014) Acceptability of smartphone application-based HIV prevention among young men who have sex with men. *AIDS and Behavior* 18 (2): 285–296.

Khoury S (2018) Online dating: breaking the taboo in conservative cultures. *Medium*, 13 December. Retrieved from https://medium.com/datadriveninvestor/online-dating-history-future-and-breaking-the-taboo-in-conservative-countries-79a959105b33 (accessed 24 July 2020).

Kjellson L (2016) Tinder and Grindr linked to more than 500 crimes, figures show. *The Telegraph*, 31 December. Retrieved from www.telegraph.co.uk/news/2016/12/31/tinder-grindr-linked-500-crimes-figures-show (accessed 29 July 2020).

Lehmiller JJ, Garcia JR, Gesselman AN and Mark, KP (2020) Less sex, but more sexual diversity: changes in sexual behavior during the COVID-19 coronavirus pandemic. *Leisure Sciences*. Epub ahead of print.

Licoppe C, Rivière CA and Morel J (2016) Grindr casual hook-ups as interactional achievements. *New Media & Society* 18 (11): 2540–2558.

Light, B, Burgess, J and Duguay S (2018) The walkthrough method: an approach to the study of apps. *New Media & Society* 20 (3): 881–900.

Lupton D (2014) Beyond techno-utopia: critical approaches to digital health technologies. *Societies* 4: 706–711.

Lupton D (2017) *Digital Health: Critical and Cross-disciplinary Perspectives*. New York: Routledge.

Mowlabocus S, Haslop C and Dasgupta R (2016) From scene to screen: the challenges and opportunities that digital platforms pose for HIV prevention work with MSM. *Social Media+ Society* 2 (4). Retrieved from https://journals.sagepub.com/doi/full/10.1177/2056305116672886 (accessed 11 January 2021).

Petrychyn J (2020) Masturbating to remain (close to) the same: sexually explicit media as habitual media. *Leisure Sciences*. Epub ahead of print.

Race K (2015) 'Party and play': online hook-up devices and the emergence of PNP practices among gay men. *Sexualities* 18 (3): 253–275.

Shapiro GK, Tatar O, Sutton A, Fisher W, Naz A, Perez S and Rosberger Z (2017) Correlates of Tinder use and risky sexual behaviours in young adults. *Cyberpsychology, Behavior, and Social Networking* 20 (12): 727–734.

Thompson R, Joy P, Numer M and Holmes D (2019) Gay men's sexual health promotion in virtual space: exploring stakeholders' attitudes and approaches to outreach on mobile apps in Nova Scotia. *The International Journal of Community Diversity* 18 (3–4):17–29.

Turban J (2018) We need to talk about how Grindr is affecting gay men's mental health. *Vox*, 4 April. Retrieved from www.vox.com/science-and-health/2018/4/4/17177058/grindr-gay-men-mental-health-psychiatrist (accessed 24 July 2020).

Wilken R, Burgess J and Albury K (2019) Dating apps and data markets: a political economy of communication approach. *Computational Culture* 7. Retrieved from http://computationalculture.net/dating-apps-and-data-markets-a-political-economy-of-communication-approach (accessed 17 November 2019).

8

'UNHOME' SWEET HOME

The construction of new normalities in Italy during COVID-19

Veronica Moretti and Antonio Maturo

Introduction

In Italy, the initial escalation of COVID-19 proved to be fiercer and more severe than in most other European countries. According to media reports, the genesis of the pandemic began on 23 January 2020, when two Chinese tourists landed at the airport of Milano Malpensa for a tour in Italy. Both were subsequently hospitalised in Rome in a critical condition, where they tested positive once the SARS-CoV-2 virus test was administered. Things then deteriorated quickly. In less than a month (21 February), 11 municipalities in northern Italy (most of them in Lombardy) were identified as the centres of the main Italian cluster, confined under quarantine and labelled as 'red zones'. By the second week of March, the whole of Italy was under lockdown after the decree to stay at home (*Io Resto a Casa*) was announced by the Prime Minister on 9 March. COVID disrupted everyday life for the population. Everyday life provides that reservoir of meanings which allows us to make sense of reality. It is the 'taken-for-granted' dimension of our existence. With this in mind, in this chapter we investigate the 'new normalities' of life in lockdown, drawing on 20 in-depth interviews we conducted with a group of childless, highly educated young adults living in northern Italy.

Journalists have often presented COVID and the consequent lockdown as an enormous 'social experiment'. Indeed, in most countries worldwide, many dimensions of everyday life have been so modified as to seem examples out of a sociology textbook. Above all, measures responding to fear of contagion – and particularly the use of face masks and social distancing – have changed interaction rituals. At least during the first weeks of lockdown in our locale, we stopped speaking with neighbours. On the few occasions we went out, we crossed the street rather than pass another person. In concealing smiles and facial expressions from sight, face masks drastically reduced metacommunication (Goffman, 1959;

Bateson, 1972), simplifying and diminishing verbal communications. Those who failed to respect restrictions related to maintaining physical distance from others – renamed 'social distancing' – provoked embarrassment and frequent outbursts of anger from people nearby, almost as if they were performing an ethnomethodology experiment (Garfinkel, 1967).

These profound changes have required us to engage our socio-semiotic abilities in analysing media content, and even dust off Susan Sontag's theories about metaphors (Sontag, 1978). We read that authorities 'hunt down the infected,' that doctors valiantly 'fight' the virus 'like heroes', that victims 'courageously succumb', that a desperate search is on for a 'weapon' against COVID. With contact-tracing apps, we enter Foucault's (1975) dimension of surveillance and the panopticon. It is no coincidence that, in this period, references to the most sociological work of fiction ever written – George Orwell's *1984* – are skyrocketing. Discussions of tracing apps often refer to the sociological perspective of network analysis (Christakis, 2009).

Thus, the first sociological concept to guide our research is that of everyday life, and the second is that of societal disruption. Numerous authors have founded sociological theories on the concept of everyday life, including Schütz (1967), Goffman (1959), Garfinkel (1967), Berger and Luckmann (1972) and Habermas (1987). We can broadly distinguish between two closely-linked characteristics of everyday life. These characteristics can be defined as the cognitive and semantic aspects of the lifeworld. The cognitive aspect of the lifeworld concerns its predictability. The reality of everyday life is self-evident and normal. Daily life is lived as if it were a natural and non-problematic social reality (Schütz, 1967). It is the *hic et nunc* reality, organised around the 'here' (*hic*) of our bodies and 'now' (*nunc*) of our present (Berger and Luckmann, 1972). We can doubt the solidity of our everyday life only in exceptional moments, for example while practising religious or metaphysical meditation (Berger and Luckmann, 1972). In all other cases, doubts about the solidity of the lifeworld are 'suspended' (Berger and Luckmann, 1972).

The cognitive dimension of everyday life also produces a semantic effect. The lifeworld is a reservoir of meanings, allowing us to make sense of reality (Schütz, 1967; Habermas, 1987). For Schütz (1967), even scientific sense is founded on the common sense of everyday life. That everyday life is a predictable, natural, immediately comprehensible world, and at the same time the basis for understanding new phenomena, does not, however, imply that it is a simple world. Indeed, Goffman (1959) has shown how face-to-face interactions – one of the principal components of everyday life – are regulated by rituals, social norms and expectations that are quite complicated and structured. Goffman analyses social interactions, demonstrating how maintaining a common definition of a situation requires great effort on the part of participants.

Garfinkel (1967) brings Goffman's propositions to extreme consequences. His breaching experiments show how social interactions are founded on tacit assumptions that are taken for granted. When these assumptions are brought to light and contradicted, subjects experience confusion at the cognitive level and anger at the moral one. Garfinkel required his students to carry out a famous example of a breaching experiment: behave like strangers at home with their own parents. After all, the home and domestic sphere are the most concrete examples of everyday life. As Rita Felski writes, invoking the theories of Agnes Heller:

> Like everyday life itself, home constitutes a base, a taken-for-granted grounding, which allows us to make forays into other worlds. It is central to the anthropomorphic organization of space in everyday life; we experience space not according to the distanced gaze of the cartographer, but in circles of increasing proximity or distance from the experiencing self. Home lies at the center of these circles. According to Heller, familiarity is an everyday need, and familiarity combines with the promise of protection and warmth to create the positive everyday associations of home.
>
> *(Felski, 2000: 85)*

During the major lockdown in Italy in the early months of the COVID pandemic, our homes were a refuge but also a prison, a place of rest but also of work. We sought to transfer the leisure activities that generally occur outside, in cafes and piazzas, to the home. Activity in the home was often frenetic: play with small children, helping older children with their homework, remote working, taking turns at the computer and exercising. Outside the home, a surreal silence reigned, broken only by ambulance sirens. We thus had to reinvent a domestic life (De Certeau, 1984) marred by hybridisation, contradiction and ambiguity.

Given the suddenness of the announcement of this lockdown, this crucial redefinition was abrupt. The lockdown was disruptive at the cognitive level. It was almost like an unexpected and fatal diagnosis for the whole of society. COVID impacted everyone, though not in a democratic way. We know that the effects of the COVID crisis are strongly linked to socioeconomic status. For this reason, we also speak of societal disruption, the second concept we use to analyse the lockdown experience. The notion of societal disruption originated in the concept of biographical disruption, the upheaval in cognitive categories that follows diagnosis of a chronic disease (Bury, 1982). This originated as an extension of the concept of biographical disruption. Michael Bury formulated the concept in one of the most cited articles in health sociology, 'Chronic illness as biographical disruption' (Bury, 1982). Starting from the analysis of semi-structured interviews administered to rheumatoid arthritis patients, Bury highlighted the explosive impact of this disease on a wide range of personal and social situations, underscoring the material, cognitive and social resources the individual must expend to confront the new situation.

> My contention is that illness, and especially chronic illness, is precisely that kind of experience where the structures of everyday life and the forms of knowledge which underpin them are disrupted. Chronic illness involves a recognition of the worlds of pain and suffering, possibly even of death, which are normally only seen as distant possibilities or the plight of others.
>
> *(Bury, 1982: 169)*

Under the impact of COVID, the lifeworld suddenly crumbled. In its place appeared what the media termed 'new normality', composed of previously unknown elements: face masks, social distancing, mortality statistics, latex gloves, house clothes and other clothes to go out shopping, disinfectants. Using semiotic terminology, we can consider them 'actants' that imposed new practices, different courses of action and novel cognitive frames.

Time, space and domestic habits

In describing the re-creation of a new normality, we took inspiration from Rita Felski's tripartition (Felski 2000), which defines daily life based upon three key aspects: time, space and modality (domestic habits). The time marking our days refers to the repetition of events, the reliable and punctual sequence characterising our activities. Space is anchored in a 'sense of home', the familiarity that certain environments – both physical and social – present to our view. Finally, modality reflects our way of life and experimentation with new habits acquired across time. This tripartition provided the starting point for data collection and the request of event narratives from our respondents.

Inspired by grounded theory, we employed the episodic narrative interview technique (Mueller, 2019) and asked participants to share stories and episodes from their everyday experiences. This method enables researchers to collect stories about an individual's life experience that can then be combined to create a coherent narrative. We were interested in stimulating participants' narrative orientation to their individual experiences of domestic life. Using snowball sampling, and in line with the purpose of 'theoretical saturation', according to which no new data appear and all concepts of the theory are well developed (Morse, 1995), we conducted 20 episodic narrative interviews with childless, highly educated adults (11 women and 9 men; 29–36 years old) living in northern Italy, the epicentre of the epidemic.

Table 8.1 provides some sociodemographic characteristics of each participant – their age, gender, marital status and their occupation. The decision to exclude individuals with children derived from the fact that daily life with children is dramatically different from that of adults able to manage their own activities in autonomy, taking into consideration only their schedule (or that of a partner). Interviewing young (under age 40) and highly educated individuals also ensured a relatively less vulnerable group compared to others in the population. Given the social distance restrictions, we conducted our interviews via Skype.

We recorded and transcribed these 'small stories' (Georgakopoulou, 2007) verbatim, comparing and synthesising the narratives into 'a chain of relevant situations' (Flick, 2000: 81). We employed thematic analysis to understand and interpret our data (Brewer, 2003). Using the Nvivo12 application, we coded each characteristic of a text and inductively developed categories through a process of constant comparison (Charmaz, 2003). The following sections describe the three dimensions evident in the participants' accounts: time, space and domestic habits.

TABLE 8.1 Sociodemographic profile of participants

Participant	*Gender*	*Age*	*Level of education*	*Marital status*	*Occupation*
01	F	34	PhD	Involved in a relationship (living together during COVID-19)	Third sector
02	F	33	Master's degree	Married (living together during COVID-19)	High school teacher
03	F	31	Master's degree	Involved in a relationship (living together during COVID-19)	Internship
04	F	31	Bachelor's degree	Involved in a relationship	Unemployed at the moment
05	F	30	PhD	Involved in a relationship	Unemployed at the moment
06	F	30	Bachelor's degree	Involved in a relationship	Tourism
07	F	32	High-school diploma	Single	Student (University)
08	M	29	Master's degree	Involved in a relationship (living together during COVID-19)	Lawyer
09	M	29	Bachelor's degree	Involved in a relationship (living together during COVID-19)	Show business
10	F	34	Master's degree	Involved in a relationship (living together during COVID-19)	High school teacher
11	F	31	Master's degree	Single	ICT
12	M	32	Master's degree	Involved in a relationship	Trade sector
13	M	36	Master's degree	Single	Unemployed at the moment
14	M	30	High-school diploma	Single	Logistical sector
15	M	29	Master's degree	Single	Graduate student
16	M	35	Bachelor's degree	Involved in a relationship (living together during COVID-19)	Show business
17	F	30	Master's degree	Single	Social services
18	M	32	PhD	Single	Communica-tion
19	M	32	Bachelor's degree	Single	Shop assistant
20	M	35	Bachelor's degree	Involved in a relationship	Social service

Time

In his development of a systematic sociology of social acceleration, Rosa (2010) draws upon the philosopher Lübbe's concept of *contraction of the present* to explain the feeling that the past no longer matters and the future has yet to count. In the present, the space of experience and horizon of expectation coincide. During the lockdown, the present seemed like the only available time frame. Especially in the first few weeks, participants learned to reject plans (from summer vacations to their futures) and interrupted habits, as well as putting many activities on standby. The one available dimension – the present – was perceived in a different way. For some individuals, time understandably expanded, with the consequent impression of flowing more slowly. But a number of participants perceived a contraction of time. For them, the lockdown accelerated the pace of daily life. Excerpts from three interviews illustrate this:

> Paradoxically, I work a lot more now than before. Students often contact me by email or online, even late in the evening, from 9 to 11. Clearly I set the goal of responding to everyone so as not to leave them feeling alone. I want to provide at least some feedback to their requests, even if it's just a simple confirmation that I received the message.
>
> *(Participant 02)*

> The pace of my mental processes has accelerated. People talk about claiming back some time for themselves, but I haven't been able to yet. On the contrary, I'm thinking all the time and not optimistically. 'Slow actions but fast thoughts.' You're always in contact with someone, so it's not like you have time to … you're always anxious to be doing something … to fill the time, and it makes you even more anxious. Time … I want to preserve some brain activity. This is not relaxing.
>
> *(Participant 04)*

> By now the weekend seems like the rest of the week with how time passes, because the days are blurring together more and more. Especially during the last two weekends, I spent practically a day and a half cleaning.
>
> *(Participant 08)*

On the other hand, other participants described the enforced slowdown as pushing them to reflect on their pre-COVID lives:

> I thought after my career was established, I would get married and have kids. But now I don't see things so rigidly. My life experience has taught me that there aren't always rules, one thing has to happen after another and sometimes the order gets reversed. Now I don't know, I'm a bit confused and maybe all this time I have to think … I don't know, maybe it will help me figure out what I want.
>
> *(Participant 10)*

This appears in line with the deep uncertainty that characterised the unprecedented lockdown situation as lived by the Italian people. Some events can radically change our lives, deeply altering the way society functions and the individual sense of security in establishing norms and routines, disrupting the stability of the identity and the *biographical continuity* of a whole nation (Giddens, 1990). As several participants noted, thinking of the future is frustrating, even distressing, as exemplified in the following quotes:

> My main goal right now is to think about my future as little as possible. This situation has truly upset every balance. I'm afraid that despite all the reflections it gives rise to, all the things you can think about in this situation, I don't know how long it will take for things to get better. Let's hope they will anyway.
>
> *(Participant 11)*

> Usually when I go to bed worn out at night, I feel like I accomplished something that day. In this case, I don't even feel like going to bed and sleeping. So the day that just ended seems pointless because I can't see the future.
>
> *(Participant 03)*

Space

The lockdown modified the geography of our homes. In parallel with how we defined everyday life – the things we take for granted 'ontologically' (Giddens, 1990) because they are fixed, almost unchanging – participants described homes that were transformed by the lockdown. The house itself was unaltered; rather, the way participants used and lived in it changed. Domestic habits and daily practices changed:

> Home … gets a little old! So there's love and hate, actually. It looks prettier, but you can't wait to leave.
>
> *(Participant 01)*

> I transformed my living room into everything I need, from the kitchen, the desk where I work, study and waste time. There's the TV next to the couch too. I don't really move around, basically I just circle around myself in this room.
>
> *(Participant 14)*

Clearly, the lockdown resulted in a renegotiation of space and reinterpretation of how objects were used. As one participant eloquently put it, such renegotiation resulted in 'a kind of task pollution':

> For example, when we're both home, I have to work remotely at the table in the living room. He rests on the couch. I experience this as a kind of task pollution. He's relaxing on the couch but I'm there working, so he can't turn

> up the volume on the TV, for example. The two things together clash, they can't coexist in the same moment.
>
> *(Participant 03)*

Similarly, other participants described the negotiations that were required:

> The freedom to be able to make a call, maybe one of us arranges with the other to go out. Or you have to go out, in general … for privacy, so as not to disturb the other one who's working. Space is a factor that impacts us because obviously when you don't have a large house, the two of you are in close contact all day.
>
> *(Participant 10)*

> As soon as we start working after breakfast, one of us stays in one room and the other in a different one. We're separated from each other until noon, until lunch time. Even if I have to pass by the kitchen, where she is, to get to the bathroom. We tend not to talk, we don't interfere with whatever the other is working on.
>
> *(Participant 01)*

New objects, new obligations and new practices shaped everyday lives, rendering once extraordinary activities mundane. Participants described having been forced to train themselves for this new context, engaging with a complex assemblage of which they were part. This sociomaterial assemblage (Lupton, 2018) was composed of objects, user instructions, but also emotions and ideas: face masks, up-to-date self-certifications, latex gloves, liquid disinfectants, good hygiene, ways of separating indoor from outdoor clothing, skills to maintain social distancing:

> I buy all my groceries for the week in one trip, usually on Wednesday – the day I've set aside for this task. So when I have to get ready to leave the house and go do this, I get anxious about a bunch of things like bringing my self-certification, putting on a face mask etc.
>
> *(Participant 19)*

The home was viewed with ambivalence. At first glance, it appears a refuge and the outside world is viewed as a 'trap' or hostile environment, as stated by one of the participants (08). Yet, as may be expected, the home becomes suffocating as well, as reported by participant number 18:

> [The outside] is a trap! The supermarket and pharmacy are right here, and so is the tobacconist.
>
> *(Participant 08)*

> I absolutely don't see [my home] as a prison, I haven't gotten to that point yet. But inevitably it's changed, without me even reflecting upon the change in how I perceive it. Before it was a refuge. After an entire day out, I immediately felt

> relaxed and wanted to rest. Now it's become practically my only living environment. So I don't see it as a prison yet, but I realise all the same that my terms of comparison with the outside world have become confused.
>
> *(Participant 18)*

Routines as a reaction to the fear of the void

For many participants, their time at home was intensely busy. The day was reorganised in a Tayloristic way to increase productivity. Taylorism is a known concept that originated from the late 1880s and early 1900s in the organisational studies sector, and it indicates the effort to use precise scientific planning for rendering the most rational and efficient work environment possible (Taylor, 1911). While this concept is now an assumed feature of economic activity, it is not an essential component of the domestic life. At home, people are usually allowed to relax and unwind without pursuing specific aims. However, during the lockdown, several individuals organised the pace of their days scientifically, allocating time for work, fitness, cooking, finding information, and so on. Not only did domestic time acquire a functional shape, but also domestic space, which was reorganised to spur productivity.

As our participants observed, there was no longer a distinction between weekdays and the weekend: both were dedicated to work. Additionally, the availability of digital technologies for working remotely served to expand time spent on work, as reported by many participants:

> I worked practically 11 hours a day, I didn't want to spend time thinking about what was happening to me.
>
> *(Participant 15)*

> So in the morning I get up at the same time as when I used to go to work. I work remotely, trying to follow more or less the same schedule as when I worked at the office.
>
> *(Participant 13)*

> I've always been pretty dependent on work. Being at home and working remotely has definitely reinforced this tendency.
>
> *(Participant 8)*

In addition, physical fitness became a fairly constant concern for participants. They understood early on that weeks, even months, spent at home would bring on weight gain and a loss of physical fitness if they did not make an effort to engage in new exercise activities from home:

> In terms of completely new things, I started jumping on a trampoline, which I never did when I went to the gym and used all the equipment there. I didn't

> feel like going out to jog, but I wanted to stay fit and agile … and this seemed like the best activity to try. I'd never done it before.
>
> *(Participant 08)*

> We try to exercise every day, something I'd never done before.
>
> *(Participant 17)*

Our group of participants stated they were drinking less than usual during the lockdown because they could no longer go out to drink while socialising with friends:

> I'm drinking a lot less, a beer every once in a while. I opened a bottle of whisky but just take sips from it. I smoke a cigarette and think about being out with my friends. It's a small way of pampering myself. But I don't feel this need. I've reduced my weekly alcohol consumption by 80 per cent.
>
> *(Participant 14)*

> I drink less. I don't drink alone. My girlfriend doesn't drink at all, so she definitely drinks less.
>
> *(Participant 09)*

Aside from their importance for mental balance, a clean house and the act of cleaning seem part of an apotropaic ritual to ward off the virus. Cleaning, disinfecting and lathering with soap are material processes, symbolic of decontamination:

> I try to be up and active by 8.30 at the latest. I don't want to lose the daily routine I've been striving to maintain.
>
> *(Participant 02)*

> I don't want to change my habits too much right now unless it's necessary, because I absolutely want to avoid this situation overturning my everyday routine. It's like I want to hold onto what I have and defend it, a kind of self-defence that has necessarily allowed the virus to enter into my life but without allowing it to overturn my everyday life.
>
> *(Participant 03)*

> I'm sort of always looking for chores to do around the house, I'm trying to stay busy any way I can.
>
> *(Participant 10)*

> I absolutely keep the house neater. Domestic order helps me to preserve mental order.
>
> *(Participant 07)*

Perhaps these ascetic regimes – more suited to the stereotype of northern Protestants than Mediterranean Catholics – were tied to the need to accomplish something with one's day. Filling the day with tasks means creating anchors. The house becomes a workplace and – when one is not working – the object of domestic labour. We clean as if it were a job responsibility.

Conclusion

In Italy, the lockdown forced us to live confined to our homes for several months. We were home at unusual times. We worked and studied at home, while our social interactions moved online. We experienced the home in a radically different way, putting it to new uses and with a new geography. The lockdown helped us understand the fragile and precarious nature of the tacit assumptions built into daily life. The frenetic activities of domestic life took place in a surreal environment. The few times we went out for trips to the grocery store or just when we watched from our windows, we felt the slowness of the urban landscape: no traffic, no noise, and fresh air in an incredibly quiet atmosphere. The stillness of eternal Sunday.

Our everyday life had been turned upside down – to quote a popular song by Diana Ross – and become our new normality. The familiar became strange and hostile, forcing us to become accustomed to a new set of obligations and habits that would have been considered bizarre prior to COVID. Participants were suddenly thrown into a situation of *anomie*, derived from the Ancient Greek word for 'lawlessness'; a situation without procedures, norms or even rituals (Durkheim, 1952 [1897]). It could be concluded they were reacting to the *horror vacui*, 'fear of the void', produced by the lockdown. In visual art, the *horror vacui* is the filling of the entire surface of a space or artwork with detail (Pawlak, 2015). In our view, some of these situations can be interpreted through the lens of *unheimlich*, the uncanny. The concept is psychoanalytical in origin, proposed by Freud (2003 [1919]). Anneleen Masschelein (2011) describes the underlying principle of the uncanny as the feeling of unease that arises when something familiar suddenly becomes strange and unfamiliar. Masschelein notes in her analysis that the concept is linked to peculiar linguistic features:

> Freud was the first to draw attention to the lexical ambivalence of the word: 'unheimlich' is the negation of 'heimlich' in the sense of 'familiar, homely', but it also coincides with the second meaning of 'heimlich' (that is) 'hidden, furtive'.
>
> *(Masschelein, 2011: 4)*

With COVID, something (very) familiar like everyday life became suddenly hostile and incomprehensible. We avoided our neighbours, visited the grocery store as infrequently as possible, and felt irritated when others walked too near. We underwent a social disruption requiring new cognitive categories, new social practices and new habits. Our experience of the domestic sphere turned ambivalent. On the one hand, it became a sure refuge and demarcation line separating us from the 'contaminated' outside world. On the other, it evolved into something of a prison and – paradoxically – a strictly regulated place; cleaning rules, but also norms of cohabitation and coexistence with the self, rituals and habits to make sense of the new reality. We filled our days with tasks, seeking to maintain a distinction between various activities. Yet often there was no difference between workdays and the weekend. We were struck by 'strange' sensations like those recounted by our participants: having to stay home on gorgeous days, drinking fine wines while listening to catastrophic news reports, participating in online *aperitivi* (having wine or other alcoholic drinks online with friends before dinner) that suddenly ended with a click, leaving us to our solitude.

Acknowledgements

While this chapter is the result of several discussions between the authors, Veronica Moretti has written the 'Time, space and domestic habits' section, and Antonio Maturo has written the 'Introduction' and 'Conclusion' sections.

References

Bateson G (1972) *Steps to an Ecology of Mind.* San Francisco, CA: Chandler Publishing Company.

Berger P and Luckmann T (1972) *The Social Construction of Reality.* Harmondsworth: Penguin.

Brewer J (2003) Content analysis. In: Miller RL and Brewer JD (eds) *The A–Z of Social Research.* London: Sage, pp. 43–45.

Bury M (1982) Chronic illness as biographical disruption. *Sociology of Health & Illness*, 4 (2): 167–182.

Charmaz K (2003) Grounded theory: objectivist and constructivist methods. In: Denzin NK and Lincoln YS (eds) *Strategies of Qualitative Inquiry.* Thousand Oaks, CA: Sage, pp. 249–291.

Christakis N (2009) *Connected: The Surprising Power of Our Social Networks and How They Shape Our Lives.* Boston, MA: Little Brown & Co.

De Certeau M (1984) *The Practice of Everyday Life.* Minneapolis: University of Minnesota Press.

Durkheim É (1952 [1897]) *Suicide: A Study in Sociology.* New York: Routledge.

Felski R (2000) *Doing Time: Feminist Theory and Postmodern Culture.* New York: NYU Press.

Flick U (2000) Episodic interviewing. In: Bauer MW and Gaskell G (eds) *Qualitative Researching with Text, Image and Sound.* London: Sage, pp. 75–92.

Foucault M (1975) *Surveiller et Punir: Naissance de la Prison.* Paris: Gallimard.

Freud S (2003 [1919]) *The Uncanny.* London: Penguin Books.

Garfinkel H (1967) *Studies in Ethnomethodology.* Englewood Cliffs, NJ: Prentice-Hall.

Georgakopoulou A (2007) Thinking big with small stories in narrative and identity analysis. In: Bamberg M (ed.), *Narrative. State of the Art.* Amsterdam: John Benjamins, pp. 146–154.

Giddens A (1990) *The Consequences of Modernity.* Cambridge: Polity Press.

Goffman E (1959) *The Presentation of Self in Everyday Life.* New York: Doubleday.

Habermas J (1987) *Lifeworld and System: A Critique of Functionalist Reason.* Boston: Beacon Press.

Lübbe H (2009) The contraction of the present. In: Rosa H and Scheuerman WE (eds) *High-Speed Society: Social Acceleration, Power and Modernity.* University Park, PA: Pennsylvania State University Press, pp. 159–179.

Lupton D (2018) *Digital Health: Critical and Cross-disciplinary Perspectives*. London: Routledge.
Masschelein A (2011) *The Unconcept: The Freudian Uncanny in Late-Twentieth-Century Theory*. Albany, NY: SUNY Press.
Morse JM (1995) The significance of saturation. *Qualitative Health Research*, 5 (2): 147–149.
Mueller RA (2019) Episodic narrative interview: capturing stories of experience with a methods fusion. *International Journal of Qualitative Methods* 18: 1–11.
Pawlak M (2015) From sociological vacuum to horror vacui: how Stefan Nowak's thesis is used in analysis of Polish society. *Polish Sociological Review* 189: 5–27.
Rosa H (2010) *Alienation and Acceleration: Towards a Critical Theory of Late-modern Temporality*. Singapore: NUS Press.
Schütz A (1967) *Collected Papers*. The Hague: Martinus Nijhoff.
Sontag S (1978) *Illness as Metaphor*. New York: Farrar, Straus and Giroux.
Taylor F (1911) *The Principles of Scientific Management*. New York: Harper.

9

QUEER AND CRIP TEMPORALITIES DURING COVID-19

Sexual practices, risk and responsibility

Ryan Thorneycroft and Lucy Nicholas

Introduction

> Today I have a message for young people: you are not invincible. This virus could put you in hospital for weeks – or even kill you. Even if you don't get sick, the choices you make about where you go could be the difference between life and death for someone else.
>
> *(World Health Organization, 2020)*

I (Ryan) am 29 years old, and I first read these words from Tedros Adhanom, director-general of the World Health Organization, on a mild autumnal Saturday morning. The night before I engaged in casual bareback (condom-free) sex with two other young men – a classically clichéd Friday night for a young gay man in Sydney's inner-city gay ghetto of Surry Hills. At the time, COVID-19 had reared its head in Australia, but we didn't know then how serious the problem was going to be. Instagram messages were exchanged and questions asked – 'have you been isolating?' and 'are you healthy?' – indicating some degree of trepidation. We all reported good health, didn't think we had too much to worry about, but perhaps most importantly, we were horny. Much has been said in the annals of academic literature about the transgressive appeal of risky sex (see Halperin, 2007; Race, 2003, 2010, 2018; Warner, 1995, 1999). So, with a degree of calculated risk, we all met at my place and fucked.

The next day, however, the world changed. Australia, suddenly, was in the midst of a pandemic. What was 'acceptable'[1] one day suddenly became unacceptable the next. The world we knew the night before was not the same world we had woken up to. Time didn't make sense anymore; it didn't flow the way it normally does. Time became odd, strange, queer, crip.

In this chapter, we use Ryan's story and experiences to ask a series of questions about the politics of sexual practices during the COVID pandemic. In a time of social distancing – which should otherwise be called physical or spatial distancing – people continue to engage in casual sex, and particularly within the gay community through sex-on-premises venues, beats and apps such as Grindr and Scruff (Banerjee and Nair, 2020; Thomas, 2020). We are interested in these practices given the material (and potentially deadly) consequences that this may have on certain populations, and we seek to reflect on the questions of risk, responsibility, deviance and desire. We invoke the concept of 'responsibilisation' (a symptom and outcome of neoliberalism) to signify the ways in which individual subjects are rendered responsible for practices that would otherwise be the duty of collective others (or historically no individual at all) (see Rose, 1996, 2007).

This approach aligns with a crip and queer theory and politics that imagines realities and futurities in new and different ways (Ramlow, 2016), and seeks to rebut the normalising effects of gay and lesbian and disability studies through modes of (radical) subversion and deconstruction (Jagose, 1996; McRuer, 2006). While responsibilisation discourses are traditionally heteronormative and ableist (Race, 2018), as well as assuming individualistic agency while invoking a responsible sociality, we suggest that COVID has cripped and queered responsibility and time. This has made crip and queer perspectives and experiences more central, and more universally experienced, providing the opportunity to imagine alternatives of a 'new future' for everyone, and to reimagine sexual practices and ethics. Thus, we use the crisis of COVID as an opportunity to rewrite crip/queer times, futures, cultures, responsibilities and sexual practices.

This essay starts by asking the question: can we criticise queer subjects for engaging in physical casual sex during the pandemic, and how can we understand its continuation without demonising it? In tackling this question, we note the ways in which some forms of sexual practices (casual queer sex) are usually demonised more than others (heteronormative/ heterosexual/monogamous sex) (Rubin, 1984). As evidenced by continued community transmission in many parts of the world, many people have made social distancing lapses (Boseley, 2020), yet there is something about (non-normative) sexuality and sexual practices that intensify notions of responsibility and apportioning blame. Queer casual sex during the COVID pandemic can be constituted as a maddening act (Thorneycroft, 2020a), yet rather than understand this phenomenon in a negative (and pathological) sense, we suggest that there are historical legacies that inform and explain such practices. We then suggest that queer sex sits at the intersections of crip/queer practice, and we move to contextualise our current moment through the lens of crip/queer times, allowing us to open up new sexual cultures and to diversify the range of practices and pleasures to *all* people. In the place of queer casual sex, we introduce forms of (crip/queer) isolation sex as an efficacious alternative, and in so doing, work to identify news forms of cultures and possibilities available during and after the COVID pandemic. In particular, we hope that this moment allows for a reconceptualising of responsibility and ethical sex away from their pervasive normative foundations, towards instead a (queer) sexual ethics focused on pleasure, and a (crip) responsibility not bound up in individualism, but focused on considering the other.

Queer sexual practices during COVID: the politics of responsibility

> Sex is presumed guilty until proven innocent. Virtually all erotic behaviour is considered bad unless a specific reason to exempt it has been established.
>
> *(Rubin, 1984: 278)*

Understanding the attribution of responsibility for the spread of COVID is an inherently fraught issue. While the cause of the global COVID pandemic can be attributed to broader social and structural forces such as globalisation, neoliberalism, capitalism and population growth, it is still the case that individual subjects have been responsibilised to limit its spread. Governments around the world have mandated im/permissible conduct to suppress or eliminate transmission. Social distancing rules were implemented, many industries were shut down, international borders closed, stay-at-home orders were mandated for non-essential activities, sick people forced into self-isolation, and so on. This is exemplary of governance being achieved through the subjectifying force of responsibilisation wherein 'the state acts remotely through … "responsibilization" … by individuals who adopt a new and specific mode of governing the self' (Pyysiäinen, Halpin and Guilfoyle, 2017: 216). Many contradictions and paradoxes lay at the heart of these rules, and they are based on economic and normative/majoritarian arguments. For example, in Australia, hairdressing salons remain open because, according to the government, they provide an 'essential service'.

Given the pervasiveness of heteronormativity in society, it is perhaps not surprising to recognise that queer casual sexual practices are constituted as impermissible and aberrant behaviours. Following some push-back, for example, in many states in Australia, leaders have accepted that people can leave their homes to visit their (presumed monogamous, cisgender, heterosexual) partners (Scanlan, 2020). The framing of this is key, however. With the tacit assumption of monogamy, the NSW Police Commissioner explained that 'visits to a partner's home are allowed' under the four essential reasons – shopping, seeking or providing (medical) care, travelling to school or work, and exercise – stating: 'I would put that [visiting a partner] under care, absolutely' (in Valencich, 2020). Given that cisgender heterosexuality is presumed 'unless otherwise stated' (Swain and Cameron, 1999: 68), we suggest these rules are written for cisgender heterosexual and monogamous subjects. Neutrality has long been critiqued as a myth in a cis-heteronormative society, and the presumption and re-constitution of the normative heterosexual nuclear family has long been noted as a discursive strategy in Australian government discourse (Nicholas, 2019). Heteronormativity, if subtle and implicit, is further compounded by the categorising of sex under care, reinforcing the heterosexual fairy-tale of sex as 'universally about the expression of health, love, self-esteem, and respect' (Halperin, 2007: 62) that queer theorists have long critiqued, and that casual queer sex does not fit.

Rubin's (1984) notion of the 'charmed circle' delineates a hierarchical valuation of sexual practices that identifies which practices (in dominant heteronormative Anglo Global North cultures) are acceptable and those which are not, a hierarchy that for the most part still holds true (Jones, 2020). The inner limits signify 'good' and 'natural' forms of sexual practices (such as monogamous and heterosexual practices) while the outer limits are 'bad' and 'unnatural' (such as promiscuous and homosexual practices) (Rubin, 1984). Given the reproductive, romantic, heterosexual norm inherent to normative constructions of sexuality, it holds that queer casual sex is constituted as bad and unnatural, particularly in the midst of the COVID pandemic, as it is well-established that violence and oppression is intensified and compounded during times of social upheaval (see Agamben, 2005; Bauman, 1989; Puar, 2007). Seeing a partner for 'care' reasons is officially sanctioned, implying that casual sex that is not connected to emotion is not as core to well-being.

While many people have made social distancing lapses – overtly and covertly, consciously and unconsciously, momentarily and continuously (Wolff et al., 2020), it strikes us that normative subjects are externalised from responsibility (e.g. hotel quarantine issues in Victoria, Australia), while non-normative subjects are remonstrated (e.g. Black Lives Matter protests). Even some queer commentary has rendered those flouting social distancing as 'ill-informed and irresponsible', according to one commentator, who went on to proclaim that 'not all of us are willing to put people's lives in danger for dick' (Box, 2020).

Ledin (2020: n.p.) notes that many gay men have continued to engage in casual gay sex to 'maintain a sense of "normalcy" in a time(s) of uncertainty'. It is important to acknowledge that casual sexual practices help maintain emotional and mental health for many (queer) populations, representing the continuation of 'experiment[ing] with the limits of … social isolation and social solidarity' key to queer sexual cultures (Halperin, 2007: 87). Permitting visits to partners for 'care'-based reasons demonstrates an implicit abjection and disavowal of other modes of sexual relationality, and potentially the ongoing taboo around discussing sexuality as a need or sexual pleasure in official discourses, with risk once again dominating sexuality discourse (Lamb, Lustig and Graling, 2013). To negate and implicitly demonise the other is to strip them of context and history.

Turning to Warner's (1995: 35) claim that '[a]bjection continues to be our dirty secret' might be one way to think through the politics of 'risky sex' and its impacts upon others – as well as to contextualise historical legacies with contemporary practices. Warner (1995), writing in the context of the HIV/AIDS crisis, wondered why he continued to engage in sex without condoms despite the (deadly) risks to himself and others. During the 1980s, HIV/AIDs was discussed with moralising terms, with claims it was caused by 'the gay life-style' and 'promiscuity' (Crimp, 1987). However, for Warner, the continued practice of sex without condoms was a seemingly ungovernable impulse he described thus: 'I recoiled so much from what I had done that it seemed to be not my choice at all. A mystery, I thought. A monster did it' (Warner, 1995: 33). Warner draws upon the 'imagery of demonic possession as a way of getting around the paradox of unintentional intention' (Halperin, 2007: 62). Warner's phenomenological and demonological description also points to what many gay men knew at the time: existing sex education policies around safe sex and celibacy were ineffectual; sex is not universally about those things in the centre of Rubin's 'charmed circle' – the expression of health, love, self-esteem and respect; and, finally, there are anti-social impulses that drive many to have sex (Crimp, 1987; Halperin, 2007; Rubin, 1984). This is what led Warner to claim that '[a]bjection continues to be our dirty secret'.

Halperin understands Warner's assertion to be about

> what it means to have someone's dick up our butts or to have someone come in our mouths. We need to admit our pleasure in being the lowest of the low, in being bad, in being outlaws, in betraying both our own values and those of the people around us. And we need to do so non-judgmentally, without having to berate ourselves for a weak ego, for a lack of self-esteem, or for some other kind of distinctively *psychological* failure.
>
> *(Halperin, 2007: 65; emphasis in the original)*

Both Warner and Halperin perfectly capture the tantalisingly transgressive appeal of risky sex, and the extent to which the 'choices' made by same-sex attracted men and the constitution of the erotic and desire cannot be divorced from the social and historical context of abjection in which it has to be understood. The internalisation of abjection and the pleasure of this in sexuality experienced by women in a culture of patriarchy has long been theorised (Irigaray, 1985), and can be extended to this analogous abjection. In a context in which gay men are already exposed to social humiliation, abjection is about taking bitter pleasure in that humiliation (Halperin, 2007). As Halperin (2007: 87) notes, abjection 'is an experiment with the limits of both destruction and survival, social isolation and social solidarity, domination and transcendence'. Sex during pandemic foregrounds the distributive nature of agency: it was not me, a monster did it.

How do we connect this account with the current pandemic, where responsibilisation is so rooted in an agentic individualistic humanism? This account illustrates the un/conscious motivations for sex, both historically and contemporarily. Queer people have an embodied familiarity with viruses given the devastation of HIV/AIDS, yet it appears neither COVID nor HIV/AIDS can stop our quest for fucking. The prospect of diminished futures is not a drastic idea for many queer subjects: the memories of the past have left mnemic traces on our bodies (see Butler, 1997). While many (young) queer people do not have the direct lived experience or memories of the HIV/AIDS pandemic, as Halperin (1995) has noted, recreational drug use and gym-junky lifestyle cultures within the queer community today operate as vectors of the past (also see Ahmed, 2002, 2004, for her comments on queer pasts and presents). Responsibility loses salience and meaning for subjects who are often only and always constituted as reckless and irresponsible because of their non-normativity. Abandoning longevity and futurity for the *here* and *now* creates alternative temporalities (Halberstam, 2005), and such temporalities can be explained through the lens of crip and queer times.

COVID and (crip/queer) time(s)

COVID has created such a disorientation in our lives that we all now live in crip and queer times. Normative time and modes of being have been de-centred and many aspects of life familiar to queers and crips have been experienced by most people. Crip and queer time challenges normative assumptions about pace and scheduling, and foregrounds different (crip and queer) temporalities by which people live (Kafer, 2013). For many people, lives have been upended; whether it be working from home or not working at all, fighting boredom at home or wrestling with an abundance of energy, imagining a post-COVID world or facing impending death, considering the limits of 'social isolation and social solidarity' (Halperin, 2007: 87), time sits differently for many. Distinct from normative (clock) time, crip and queer time points to the flexible times within which different bodies live their lives. Crip and queer time develops as a way of rejecting normative/ableist/heteronormative associations and logics, and as a way of living differently.

Crip time can be understood in many different ways, both as a site of liberation and alienation. McDonald (2020) understands crip time as extra time:

> I live by a different time to you … I have cerebral palsy, I can't walk or talk, I use an alphabet board, and I communicate at the rate of 450 words an hour compared to your 150 words in a minute – twenty times as slow. A slow world would be my heaven. I am forced to live in your world, a fast hard one. If slow rays flew from me I would be able to live in this world. I need to speed up, or you need to slow down.

McDonald (2020) notes the many ways in which her temporality is slower to others. Kafer (2013) adds to this picture by suggesting that notions of crip time as extra time are often the result of ableist and disablist barriers (such as difficult-to-access buildings, or the ableist compulsion for productivity). In response, Kafer (2013) suggests that crip time should be about flexible time and not just extra time. For example, some people who identify as autistic or mad often operate on accelerated time. Samuels (2017) also notes how crip time can result in disorientation, for herself and others: 'I look 25, feel 85, and just want to live like the other 40-somethings I know.' Synchronous normative time has the capacity to butt up against crip time.

There are significant overlaps between crip and queer time. For example, Halberstam (2005) speculates that queer time originated from the HIV/AIDS crisis. The epidemic completely upended the conventions of family, inheritance, and child-rearing, and the creation of alternative queer temporalities and socialities emerged from it. The saying 'live fast, die young [and leave a beautiful corpse]' comes to mind. Alternative subcultures are so compelling because of their capacity to open up alternative temporospatial notions and opportunities. Halberstam (2005: 2) suggests these subcultures 'produce alternative temporalities by allowing their participants to believe that their futures can be imagined according to logics that lie outside of those paradigmatic markers of life experience – namely, birth, marriage, reproduction, and death'.

Many non-queer and non-crip subjects are now experiencing a time akin to crip/queer time, with normative life trajectories on hold and a need for a freeze on futurity. Normative time, normative sex and normative (individualist) ethics are upended during COVID. Subscribing to this position, and returning to the issue of COVID and casual gay sex, we ask ourselves the following question: in this historical moment, what kind of efficacious queer sexual futures and temporalities can we (re)imagine? Specifically, in line with our scholarly, activist, and queer subject positions, how can we propose a more responsible form of sexual practices during this pandemic that simultaneously creates new crip/queer temporalities and ensures that heteronormative and ableist practices and futures can be cripped and queered? We turn to this question in the final section by proposing crip/queer forms of isolation sex.[2]

Crip/queer sexual pandemic futures

> [Q]ueer and crip activisms share a will to remake the world, given the ways in which injustice, oppression, and hierarchy are built (sometimes quite literally) into the structures of contemporary society.
>
> *(McRuer, 2012: n.p.)*

> Perhaps now is the time for us all to move out of our normative shadows and embrace our inherent potential to be non-normative. Perhaps now is time for a politics of abnormality.
>
> *(Goodley, 2014: 135)*

Sexual health advocates and professionals remain vexed on the ethics and practices of (casual) sex during this pandemic (Ledin, 2020). While some have advocated celibacy, others have noted that such practices have historically had little capital and/or effectiveness (see Berkowitz and Callen, 1983; Crimp, 1987). Thus, concepts such as 'negotiated safety' and 'practices of responsibility,' long invoked in queer contexts, have emerged as alternative practices and possibilities. Following Ledin (2020), we put forth the notion of 'isolation sex' in the hope that it might accommodate a more efficacious politics of sexual practices and pleasures during the COVID pandemic that speaks to this interplay of isolation and solidarity, or what we call sociality. Isolation sex offers the space to rethink notions of pleasure and practice, and they can be engaged in alone or with others, both virtually and physically. In putting forth this notion of isolation sex, we are not doing so with only crip and queer people in mind. In keeping with our crip/queer politics, and our broader aims of cripping ableism and queering heteronormativity, we also want to recognise the potential that isolation sex offers for abled/ableist and heteronormative/heterosexist subjects. Such a politics enables a way of being sexual, and of living otherwise during the crip/queer temporalities and spatialities we currently occupy.

Isolation sex with oneself may involve the use of sex toys and vibrators, watching pornography, making solo videos, wearing stimulating clothing, and so on. Ledin (2020) suggests that many people seek out sexual gratification from others without fully exploring their own bodies and its desires. He writes that we should

> illuminate the pleasures our bodies are capable of in an isolated space, trying and practicing – and sometimes failing! – to make sense of our own pleasures and desires, which are specific to each body. It's a trial run, of sorts, where we might remain with ourselves, seek out those pleasures we seek from others, and, if we are lucky, find those sweet spots some of us lust after but never quite find. We can find greater meaning in how we value the sexual nature of the body by using this period to self-recognise, to put forward a *self-sex politics* that makes sex both *during* and *after* COVID-19 *possible.*
>
> *(Ledin, 2020; emphasis in the original)*

Ledin's (2020) account highlights the potentialities open to individuals to explore their pleasures. Such an account works to protect others from COVID, but also, and perhaps just as importantly, to allow individuals to open up new avenues of pleasure, being and becoming. This speaks to queer reconfigurations of sexual ethics that attempt to separate sex from social values and to consider instead a 'sexual value system' (Rubin, 1984: 280) that centres maximising pleasure of both the self and the other (Nicholas, 2014). Orienting the sexual value system away from identities and social values, many development and rights discourses have theorised that the right to sexual pleasure ought to be the aim of sexuality (Jolly, 2007). This moment of 'isolation' thus offers a chance for those traditionally not abjected by the sexual value system to reflect on what sex is *for*, and what feels good.

What is key to many accounts of queer sexual ethics is that it also entails an ethical relationality to others, which could be called a responsibility. That is, one's sexual pleasure should not impede that of others and, indeed, should strive to maximise the conditions for it (Nicholas, 2014). Abandoning the normative sexual value system also rewrites who and what is sexy, 'what counts as sex' (Mollow and McRuer, 2012: 32), what desire is, and challenges notions of 'isolation', 'independence' and 'seclusion', all key concerns in a crip theory focused on sex/uality. Rethinking isolation also provides an opportunity for reflection on how pleasure can be sought with others in new ways, divorced from normative reproductive/romance paradigms.

Isolation sex with other people may occur virtually (online) or physically (with those with whom you reside) (Lehmiller et al., 2020). Virtual isolation sex with others might involve sexting, cybersex or phone-sex with friends or strangers, as well as participation in online sex forums (Petrychyn, 2020). Physically, it may involve sexual practices with those whom you live with (Ledin, 2020). The practices may be sexual pleasures that are conventional or unconventional, standard or new, experimental or traditional. The aim is to open up ways in which sexual practices can occur in less normative and more ethical frameworks, and to provide an alternative sexual health solution (Ledin, 2020).

Isolation sex provides ample crip/queer opportunities and forms of pleasure. Queer sex is already well acquainted with several practices – fisting, group sex, watersports and so on – that open up new forms of queer pleasures, cultures, and politics. So too, crip sex transforms conventional notions of sexual practice, rewrites understandings of normative sexual attraction and desire, and opens up conventional meanings of sexual practice (Mollow and McRuer, 2012). Pleasure can be understood in different ways, bodies can do different things (stumping, for example), erogenous zones can be remapped, and the emphasis on acts rather than identities helps recast the discipline of sexuality (see Thorneycroft, 2020b). The aim is to open up new sexual cultures and to diversify the range of sexual practices and pleasures open to *all* people, and COVID provides this opportunity.

Aspects of crip and queer sex force us to rethink ableist and heteronormative notions of pleasure, desires and sexual practices (see Thorneycroft, 2020b). To engage in ethical forms of queer isolation sex at this historical juncture is to protect crip and older bodies from COVID, and this means the actors are engaging in efficacious crip/queer sexual practices. Broadening rather than narrowing what we understand to be sexual practices opens up new forms of cultures and possibilities available during and after COVID. The question will be: do we want to embrace crip and queer times, and imagine more ways of living differently and otherwise into the future?

Concluding remarks: a crip and queer ethics of responsibility and sociality

The COVID pandemic has intensified notions of un/acceptable (sexual) practices. Conventional and monogamous practices are legitimated but unconventional and casual encounters are pathologised and frowned upon. Given COVID has upended many of our lives, it is important that we turn to imagining futures that we want to live in and with. It is in this regard that we have sought to use the crisis of COVID as a way of rethinking queer/crip practices and futures.

Considering the ethics of sexual cultures in turn provides the opportunity to consider the implication of crip and queer sexual ethics for wider sociality and responsibility, during and after COVID. It has long been argued that the self that is universalised (the heteronormative, abled self) is not compelled to reflect on the particularity of their position, causing a lack of empathy for and thus a demonising of 'others'. Could COVID then compel this decentring, provoking the previously centred 'to live in ways that maintain a critical and transformative relation' (Butler, 2004: 3) to normative modes of being, of sexuality, and of time and productivity? In turn, could this thus compel both reflection on the norms through which one is constituted and a real sense of responsibility or reciprocity for others abjected by these norms? This is '"queer" … more as a relational process, rather than as a simple identity category' (Brown, 2007: 2687).

From the individualised responsibility of neoliberal responses to a very social pandemic, then, queer and crip thinking can offer an ethics of responsibility that does not collapse back into atomised and ontologically naïve 'equalism'. Rather, it can account for the broader social and structural forces that have been largely absent from accounts of COVID, drawing attention to the uneven playing field that render universal mandates problematic. Alongside some intensification of abjection in responsibilisation discourses, COVID has seen some exemplary moments of social care, and a centring of the non-normative; this may well be fleeting for this exceptional moment, rather than the new rule(?).

We have meditated on the politics of 'risky sex' during this pandemic, speculated about their queer/crip orientations, imagined ourselves in crip/queer times, and sought to imagine crip/queer sexual futures. This exposition has been explorative and imaginary, holding out hope for crip/queer futures. When we are unable to match our bodies and ways of life to normative (clock) time, it is then time *for time* to better match our own bodies, practices, and ways of life. Isolation sex queers and crips heteronormative and ableist ways of thinking and doing and opens up alternative avenues and subcultures for us. Isolation sex imagines sex differently, and in so doing, orients us to different and alternative beings, doings and futures.

Notes

1 This phrase is in quotation marks to highlight the ways in which many forms of (queer) sex are always and only constituted as 'unacceptable' by some members of the community.
2 In putting forth these ideas we are indebted to the work of Chase Ledin (see https://chaseledin.com).

References

Agamben G (2005) *State of Exception*. Chicago, IL: The University of Chicago Press.

Ahmed S (2002) This other and other others. *Economy and Society* 31 (4): 558–572.

Ahmed S (2004) Collective feelings: or, the impressions left by others. *Theory, Culture & Society* 21 (2): 25–42.

Banerjee D and Nair VS (2020) 'The untold side of COVID-19': struggle and perspective of the sexual minorities. *Journal of Psychosexual Health* 2 (2): 113–120.

Bauman Z (1989) *Modernity and the Holocaust*. Cambridge: Polity Press.

Berkowitz R and Callen M (1983) *How to Have Sex during an Epidemic: One Approach*. New York: Tower Press.

Boseley M (2020) Victoria may introduce more restrictions with 1 in 4 Covid-19 cases not isolating and 627 new cases recorded. *The Guardian*, 31 July. Retrieved from www.theguardian.com/australia-news/2020/jul/31/victoria-may-introduce-more-restrictions-with-1-in-4-covid-19-cases-not-isolating-and-627-new-cases-recorded (accessed 31 July 2020).

Box B (2020) Some gays refuse to let COVID-19 keep them from hooking up. *IN Magazine*, 31 March. Retrieved from http://inmagazine.ca/2020/03/some-gays-refuse-to-let-covid-19-keep-them-from-hooking-up (accessed 4 July 2020).

Brown G (2007) Mutinous eruptions: autonomous spaces of radical queer activism. *Environment & Planning A* 39 (11): 2685–2698.

Butler J (1997) *Excitable Speech: A Politics of the Performative*. New York: Routledge.

Butler J (2004) *Undoing Gender*. New York: Routledge.
Crimp D (1987) How to have promiscuity in an epidemic. *October* 43 (Winter): 237–271.
Goodley D (2014) *Dis/ability Studies: Theorising Disablism and Ableism*. New York: Routledge.
Halberstam J (2005) *In a Queer Time and Place: Transgender Bodies, Subcultural Lives*. New York: New York University Press.
Halperin DM (1995) *Saint Foucault: Towards a Gay Hagiography*. Oxford: Oxford University Press.
Halperin DM (2007) *What Do Gay Men Want? An Essay on Sex, Risk, and Subjectivity*. Ann Arbor, MI: The University of Michigan Press.
Irigaray L (1985) *This Sex Which is Not One*, trans. Porter C and Burke C. New York: Cornell University Press.
Jagose A (1996) *Queer Theory: An Introduction*. New York: New York University Press.
Jolly S (2007) *Why the development industry should get over its obsession with bad sex and start to think about pleasure*. Institute of Development Studies (IDS) Working Paper 283, May. Brighton: University of Sussex.
Jones RL (2020) Later life sex and Rubin's 'charmed circle'. *Sexuality & Culture* 24: 1480–1498.
Kafer A (2013) *Feminist, Queer, Crip*. Bloomington, IN: Indiana University Press.
Lamb S, Lustig K, and Graling K (2013) The use and misuse of pleasure in sex education curricula. *Sex Education* 13 (3): 305–318.
Ledin C (2020) Socialising the isolation period. Retrieved from https://chaseledin.com/2020/03/23/socialising-the-isolation-period (accessed 18 May 2020).
Lehmiller JL, Garcia JR, Gesselman AN and Mark KP (2020) Less sex, but more sexual diversity: changes in sexual behavior during the COVID-19 coronavirus pandemic. *Leisure Sciences: An Interdisciplinary Journal*. Epub ahead of print.
McDonald A (2020) Crip time. Retrieved from www.annemcdonaldcentre.org.au/crip-time (accessed 15 May 2020).
McRuer R (2002) Compulsory able-bodiedness and queer/disabled existence. In: Snyder SL, Brueggemann BJ and Garland Thomson R (eds) *Disability Studies: Enabling the Humanities*. New York: The Modern Language Association of America, pp. 88–99.
McRuer R (2006) *Crip Theory: Cultural Signs of Queerness and Disability*. New York: New York University Press.
McRuer R (2012) Cripping queer politics, or the dangers of neoliberalism. *Scholar & Feminist Online* 10 (1–2). Retrieved from http://sfonline.barnard.edu/a-new-queer-agenda/cripping-queer-politics-or-the-dangers-of-neoliberalism (accessed 6 October 2020).
Mollow A and McRuer R (2012) Introduction. In: McRuer R and Mollow A (eds) *Sex and Disability*. Durham, NC: Duke University Press, pp. 1–36.
Nicholas L (2014) *Queer Post-gender Ethics: The Shape of Selves to Come*. Basingstoke: Palgrave Macmillan.
Nicholas L (2019) Whiteness, heteropaternalism and the gendered politics of settler colonial populist backlash culture in Australia. *Social Politics: International Studies in Gender, State and Society* 27 (2): 234–257.
Petrychyn J (2020) Masturbating to remain (close to) the same: sexually explicit media as habitual media. *Leisure Sciences: An Interdisciplinary Journal*. Epub ahead of print.
Puar JK (2007) *Terrorist Assemblages: Homonationalism in Queer Times*. Durham, NC: Duke University Press.
Pyysiäinen J, Halpin D and Guilfoyle A (2017) Neoliberal governance and 'responsibilization' of agents: reassessing the mechanisms of responsibility-shift in neoliberal discursive environments. *Distinktion: Journal of Social Theory* 18 (2): 215–235.
Race K (2001) The undetectable crisis: changing technologies of risk. *Sexualities* 4 (2): 167–189.

Race K (2003) Revaluation of risk among gay men. *AIDS Education and Prevention* 15 (4): 369–381.

Race K (2010) Engaging in a culture of barebacking: gay men and the risk of HIV prevention. In: Davis M and Squire C (eds) *HIV Treatment and Prevention Technologies in International Perspective*. London: Palgrave Macmillan, pp. 144–166.

Race K (2018) *The Gay Science: Intimate Experiments with the Problem of HIV*. New York: Routledge.

Ramlow TR (2016) Queering, cripping. In: Giffney N and O'Rourke M (eds) *The Ashgate Research Companion to Queer Theory*. New York: Routledge, pp. 129–146.

Rose N (1996) The death of the social? Re-figuring the territory of government. *International Journal of Human Resource Management* 25 (3): 327–356.

Rose N (2007) *The Politics of Life Itself: Biomedicine, Power, and Subjectivity in the Twenty-first Century*. Princeton, NJ: Princeton University Press.

Rubin GS (1984) Thinking sex: notes for a radical theory of the politics of sexuality. In: Vance CS (ed.) *Pleasure and Danger: Exploring Female Sexuality*. Boston, MA: Routledge and Kegan Paul, pp. 267–319.

Samuels E (2017) Six ways of looking at crip time. *Disability Studies Quarterly* 37 (3). Retrieved from https://dsq-sds.org/article/view/5824 (accessed 6 October 2020).

Scanlan R (2020) Coronavirus Australia: what are the rules about seeing my partner during self-isolation? *news.com.au*, 1 April. Retrieved from www.news.com.au/lifestyle/health/health-problems/coronavirus-australia-what-are-the-rules-about-seeing-my-partner-during-selfisolation/news-story/93bf3a8e3ac07d532c3c040c6373b6f9 (accessed 6 July 2020).

Swain J and Cameron C (1999) Unless otherwise stated: discourses of labelling and identity in coming out. In: Corker M and French S (eds) *Disability Discourse*. Buckingham: Open University Press, pp. 68–78.

Thomas S (2020) Mask use and sex on premises: navigating a COVID-19 world? *Star Observer*. Retrieved from www.starobserver.com.au/news/national-news/mask-use-sex-on-premises-navigating-a-covid-19-world/196714 (accessed 31 July 2020).

Thorneycroft R (2020a) Crip theory and mad studies: intersections and points of departure. *Canadian Journal of Disability Studies* 9 (1): 91–121.

Thorneycroft R (2020b) If not a fist, then what about a stump? Ableism and heteronormativity within Australia's porn regulations. *Porn Studies* 7 (2): 152–167.

Valencich G (2020) NSW couples cleared to visit each other's homes during coronavirus pandemic. *7 News*, 1 April. Retrieved from https://7news.com.au/lifestyle/health-wellbeing/nsw-couples-cleared-to-visit-each-others-homes-during-coronavirus-pandemic-c-946295 (accessed 4 July 2020).

Warner M (1995) Unsafe: why gay men are having risky sex. *The Village Voice*, 31 January: 33–36.

Warner M (1999) *The Trouble with Normal: Sex, Politics, and the Ethics of Queer Life*. Cambridge, MA: Harvard University Press.

Wolff W, Martarelli CS, Schüler J and Bieleke M (2020) High boredom proneness and low trait self-control impair adherence to social distancing guidelines during the COVID-19 pandemic. *International Journal of Environmental Research and Public Health* 17 (15): 5420.

World Health Organization (2020) WHO Director-General's opening remarks at the media briefing on COVID-19 – 20 March 2020. Retrieved from www.who.int/director-general/speeches/detail/who-director-general-s-opening-remarks-at-the-media-briefing-on-covid-19—20-march-2020 (accessed 4 July 2020).

10

ISOL-AID, ART AND WELLBEING

Posthuman community amid COVID-19

Marissa Willcox, Anna Hickey-Moody and Anne M. Harris

Introduction

Writing from isolated individual locations across Melbourne, we author this paper as we experience the strictest lockdown and curfew Australia has seen in 100 years. Imposed in response to a second wave of COVID-19 (which emerged for us in July 2020), the state-enforced social distancing measures have resulted in almost all social connection occurring through social media via digital devices (Fuchs, 2020). This has prompted a significant shift in the ways live art and music is accessed, as performance is now largely mediated through digital live streams. Artists are being forced into even more precarious employment conditions due to the pandemic, demanding increased resilience amid an already-uncertain gig economy (Morgan and Nelligan, 2018; Taylor and Luckman, 2020) and a national narrative which devalues the arts through ever-shrinking funding schemes (Caust, 2019, 2020). An enduring reconfiguration of sociality lingers (Fullagar and Pavlidis, 2020), as artists and audience members alike experiment with strategies for connection and, indeed, survival. However, this type of digitally mediated social connection is only available for those with the technology to support it, bringing up pre-existing issues of inequality between social classes, access and wellbeing (Robinson et al., 2020; Barber and Naepi, 2020; Bhatia, 2020).

In this chapter, we analyse a case study of the Australian Instagram Live music festival 'Isol-AID' – an artist community's response to the current pandemic. The emergence of this online festival during lockdown warrants further investigation into how the arts contribute to wellbeing[1] and whether online live performance can offer more accessibility options to arts spaces. In what follows, we consider Instagram Live and streamed performance a posthuman assemblage in order to highlight the importance of nonhuman actants (such as phones, social media platforms, Wi Fi, colours, sounds) in the production of community.

Humans are fundamentally enmeshed with, and co-constituted by, the more-than-human. We interview one of the Isol-AID creators to illustrate this link and ask how community connection through more-than-human devices and platforms can address such issues as access to the arts as a form of wellbeing. We build on literature about social prescribing to suggest that Instagram Live can facilitate engagement in forms of arts practice that are therapeutic, and therefore acts as a new digital health resource. Living physically distant in a global pandemic, there has never been a more pertinent time to recognise the importance of access to the arts as an essential component of community making, health and wellbeing.

Isol-Aid

Isol-AID describes itself as a 'socially (media) distanced music festival' in its Instagram bio. Starting in Australia to support local artists and showcase Australian performers, it has a growing international fan base. The festival operates through a stream of live performances that are broadcast through an artist's or band's Instagram Live feed. It gained over 43,000 followers in less than three months and raised tens of thousands of dollars amid a wave of artists switching to digital live performance. Running in its seventeenth week at the time of writing, Isol-AID was brought to life by Australian artists and community organisers Emily Ulman, Rhiannon Atkinson-Howatt and Shannen Egan to raise money for Support Act, a mental health non-profit organisation that provides relief funding to support Australian musicians through crisis. Taking on new artists as it continues its unprecedented success, running week after week, Isol-AID has now started accepting donations that go directly to the artists.

For us, the success of Isol-AID highlights the posthuman nature of our daily lives. There are so many ways that humans rely on nonhuman assemblages to connect in times of crisis. The concept of *access to the arts* needs to be seen as a public health measure which contributes to wellbeing (Stuckey and Nobel, 2010; Mastandrea et al., 2019). Extending the work of arts and accessibility scholars, we contend that creating more opportunities for arts-based interventions in healing and health will offer greater public health outcomes and community connection (Rogers, 1993; Camic and Chatterjee, 2013; Fleming and Whitaker, 2019). As such, the efforts of artists to create community amid isolation need to be taken into account in future arts funding and policy contexts. Exploring the cultural significance of Isol-AID, we show how Instagram and the artists involved have constructed and relied on the posthuman community assemblage of Instagram Live during a broader industry shift to digital streamed performance due to COVID.

Figure 10.1 shows the Isol-AID Instagram profile and their first gig poster. On the back of the poster is the set list and the Instagram handle of the performers (the poster is on a package of toilet paper, a comment on panic-buying during the pandemic). When it's time to perform, festival-goers log onto the artist's or band's Instagram Live feed and watch their set. The artist who performs next is

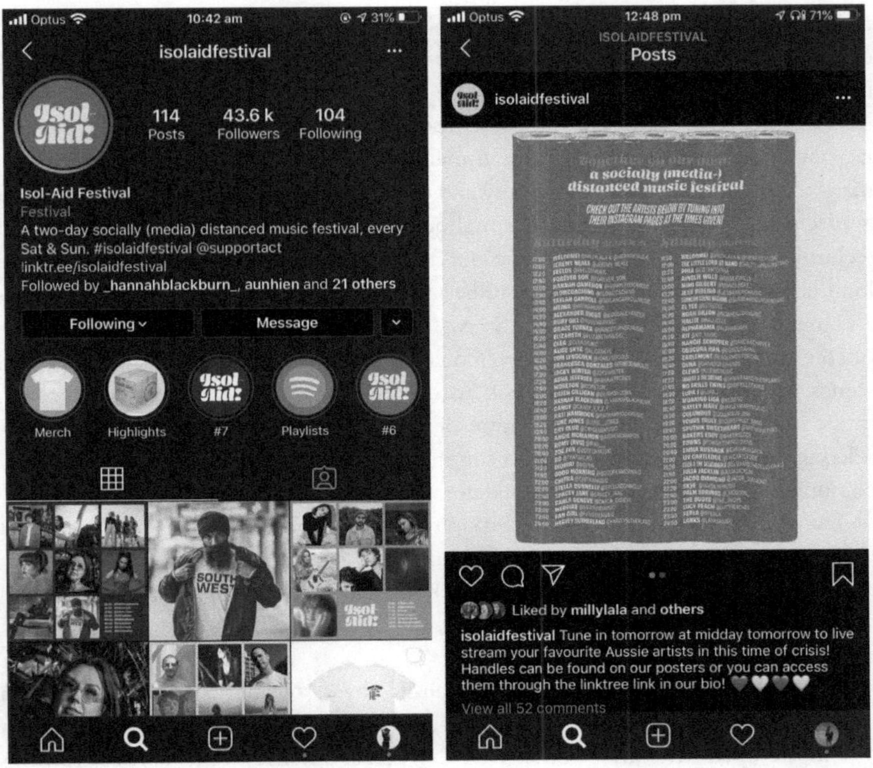

FIGURE 10.1 Isol-AID Instagram bio, band poster and set list
Source: Marissa Willcox, with permission of Rhiannon Atkinson-Howatt

then tagged in the live video and the audience moves to this artist's feed. We interviewed Rhiannon Atkinson-Howatt (@merpiremusic) for this chapter. At the time of writing, Rhiannon has stepped back from organising the event as it has grown too large for her to keep up with her own music and manage the recurring event series.

The liveness of posthuman community

Rosi Braidotti, a founding scholar of posthuman thinking, says 'as far as I'm concerned, the challenge of the posthuman condition consists in grabbing the opportunities offered by the decline of the unitary subject position upheld by humanism, which has mutated in a number of complex directions' (Braidotti, 2013: 50). Throughout her book *The Posthuman* (2013), Braidotti asks readers and scholars to think beyond the human subject as the centre of the social world. This thinking provides the opportunity to navigate hybrid and ontologically complex subjectivities and environments in ways that re-create and re-define preconceived notions of what it means to be human (or more than human). As a 'live', and continually evolving philosophy, posthumanism examines the enmeshment of technological and societal shifts in the consideration and enactment of things we thought we knew, such as gender, race, sexuality, environment and technology, and their multiple entanglements.

Our interview with Rhiannon Atkinson-Howatt about the future of digitally facilitated live community connection methods shows the importance of the more-than-human in facilitating community and calls for a rethinking of the current support available for artist communities throughout crisis. Enquiries into communities and scenes within the music industry are not new (Whiteley, 2012). Scene theory has a long history within popular music studies, which informs our discussion of musicians and musical practices (for more, see Straw, 1991; Bennett & Rogers, 2016). The types of community we are addressing here could be described as virtual and/or trans-local scenes. However, we choose to look at the ways that community is made through music making and the complex nature of technological entanglements. When considering the dimensions of arts-based communities, it is obvious that they are primarily comprised through material elements such as sound, technology, space and place.

The ability to gather together through an ever-evolving 'we' is something that exists beyond the bounds of the individual (or even collective) human. 'We' turn to more-than-human elements which help orient us towards one another, such as digital technology. Braidotti writes:

> Virtual possibilities need to be actualized, by a missing 'we', that is to say a transversal subject that will be composed in concrete historical circumstances, in the open structure of time, with the virtual potentials at its core … It is this complexity and heterogeneity that constitute posthuman subjectivity, defined as the composition of posthuman subjects who want to know otherwise and produce knowledge differently.
>
> *(Braidotti, 2019: 155)*

Braidotti's posthumanist perspective of a virtually possible 'we' recognises the agency in technology for facilitating our communities. Isol-AID is made by the capabilities of the artists, but also the liveness of digitally streamed connections. When asked why her team chose Instagram Live as their stage, Rhiannon responded by saying:

> Emily and I really wanted to be able to provide a community – a safe, supportive community for not only people that were missing out on playing gigs, but for audience members who had bought tickets, as they needed a space to grieve since they couldn't see their artists. So, it was like a double – yeah, a double community intention really.

This 'double community intention' showed that Isol-AID was needed not only for the artists to raise money, but also for the fans who had bought tickets to live shows. Rhiannon explains this community intention and the benefits of using Instagram:

> It's not only the performances themselves, but the community with other audience members talking to each other in the comments, which is another reason why we chose Instagram. Audience members could communicate in real time and talk about how excited they were that Angie (Angie McMahon) was playing for their screen right now, in her pyjamas!

The sensory engagement with performance takes on a removed yet also intimate quality. Audience members are watching alone, not rubbing against each other in the crowd; performers are dressed in pyjamas playing music from their lounge rooms; love hearts and applause emojis bombard the phone's comment stream, yet the sound of silence surrounds them after they finish their set. The simultaneously personal and public experience of performing through digital live stream is entangled with the genres of digital platforms and is notably different from the way live performances feel in physical venues.

We are talking specifically about live performance methods and not music consumption more generally. Our investigation is into the ways that the mediation of performance and community connection has changed due to COVID. While many multisensory experiences involving beer, bodies and the reverberation of soundwaves inform embodied experiences of attending a live in-person gig, a live performance online is differently mediated through the humans and technologies that form another kind of proximity. Considerations of different forms of liveness do not erase the unique aspects of each context. The famous 1990s performance studies 'liveness debate' between Peggy Phelan and Phillip Auslander has informed the scholarship on the evolving nature of live performance in increasingly mediated/mediatised cultures (Harris and Holman Jones, 2016; Diamond et al., 2017; Auslander, 2008; Phelan, 2004). For Phelan, physical proximity defines important aspects of the experience of live performance, while for Auslander the notion of 'live' cannot be binarised or claim superiority in relation to 'virtual' or 'mediatised' performance, given they emerged from different temporalities and cultural contexts.

Temporality is central to this debate, as seen in Phelan's argument that performance that is recorded and no longer happening in the present ceases to become 'live' – a claim that Instagram live streaming (and other social media platforms) challenges, 25 years on. Since the 1990s, audience and performer experiences and enactments of liveness continue to evolve, and social media has become the latest enactment of these increasingly overlapping considerations. Indeed, the promise of new materialist and posthumanist studies is to problematise the notion of liveness in new ways, moving beyond the human into more expansive understandings of animacy, the animate, and what constitutes the state of being 'alive' (Harris and Holman Jones, 2019; Chen, 2012).

Applying considerations of liveness and posthuman, or more-than-human, connectivity to post COVID communities, Nikolic and Skinner's work broadens the definition of 'we' through a discussion of what it means to make community:

> The always reassembled 'we' simply cannot not partake in material-discursive commoning-community; the question is rather that of orientation and ecology,

> of the degree of entanglement ... There is no distance between a subject and multispecies in/organic commoning-community; there are only patterns of care and their un/making.
>
> *(Nikolic and Skinner, 2019: 11–12)*

Commoning can be seen as a practice of collaborating and sharing to meet everyday needs and achieve wellbeing, of individuals, communities and lived-in environments. Community and commoning as defined by Nikolic and Skinner (2019) is a practice of people coming together, both with other people and the more-than-human, through an ethics of care, making and being with. The notion of live community connection has posthuman roots. Whether made by digital technology, music technology, faith in something, or love for someone, community is indefinitely evolving and needs to be considered not for its human or nonhumanness, but for its agency in delivering necessities like creativity, social connection and health.

Access to art as wellbeing

The shift to online performance during COVID has highlighted the possible health and wellbeing outcomes of arts access. We consider digital forms of connectivity an important method of accessing 'liveness' in performance and explore how digital and physically proximate live shows can be bridged to expand enactments of live performance to broader audiences.

Calling for a diversification of what constitutes methods of community connection, we build on the notion of social prescribing (Rogers, 1993; Kimberlee, 2015; Barker, 2019) in arguing that access to and involvement in the arts are essential to mental wellbeing and community cohesion. Richard Kimberlee explains:

> SP [social prescribing] emerged as a mechanism for linking people using primary care with support in their community ... In these services there are potential solutions to the wider determinants of mental health ... And in many ways SP is a route to reducing social exclusion.
>
> *(Kimberlee, 2015: 104–105)*

Social prescribing emerged as a method from person-centred psychology and is widely attributed to psychologist Carl Rogers. Using a feminist creative approach, Natalie Rogers (1993: 4) advanced her father's work by developing a therapeutic process called the creative connection RM, which interweaves all the expressive arts in a psychological process of healing. She recognised that the social and psychological determinants of health are largely what can limit or open pathways towards creativity. The social determinants of health are the conditions in which people are born, grow, live, work and age. These circumstances are shaped by the distribution of money, power and resources at global, national and local levels. The social determinants of health are mostly responsible for health inequities – the unfair and avoidable differences in health status seen within and between countries

(World Health Organization, 2020). They can be mediated through creative expression and social interaction. As such, access to the arts should be considered a crucial component in a community's broader overall health and wellbeing.

Isol-AID and other live musical performance methods emerging amid lockdown provide a much-needed contribution to our understanding of community connection and artistic expression. Rhiannon describes this process of connection as follows:

> This isn't stuff you can buy, because there isn't any money involved at this stage. It's just like, 'Are you struggling? Yeah, me too, let's play a live gig and talk about it and sing about it.' And it was almost like Isol-AID became a hug from a parent, being like, 'I know it's really scary right now, but we've got each other, so let's just hold each other while we have no idea what's going on, let's sing about it, and we can stay connected and work it out as we go.'

A 'hug from a parent' is exactly what Isol-AID felt like. In times of high anxiety and stress, for both the artists and audience, Barker (2019: 77) suggests that such 'creative activities can have a healing and protective effect on mental wellbeing. They can facilitate relaxation, provide a means of self-expression, reduce blood pressure, boost the immune system and reduce stress'. Supporting artists throughout this economic crisis using online or in physical venues should therefore be considered a top priority amid a global pandemic, as it contributes to community health and wellbeing.

The impacts of social prescribing

There is a growing body of UK-based research which looks at the benefits of implementing social prescribing measures and access to the arts. Stickley and Duncan (2007) investigate Nottingham's *Art in Mind*'s conceptualisation and implementation, and find that 'when attention is given to the importance of developing community networks that are designed to build social capital for participating groups and individuals, we can combat health and social inequalities' (Stickley and Duncan, 2007: 24). Later, Stickley and Hui (2012) examined the effects of art on prescription for people who often used mental health services. They found that for 'community-based arts groups … participants gained a sense of pride in their work, and experienced psychological, social and occupational benefits' (Stickley and Hui, 2012: 579). Increased creative connection among individuals builds social ties which work towards improving mental health outcomes. And, as in-person social connection is limited amid COVID, creative expression and connection through live digital platforms can serve as a measure of accessing health benefits, creating a new digital health resource.

The extensive work on social prescribing of art, in the UK specifically, points to the comparison that Jo Caust (2020) makes, which looks at how governments such as in the UK are contributing more funding to arts sectors than is Australia. Caust (2020) points out that since 2016 arts funding has decreased exponentially in Australia and amid the coronavirus lockdowns 75 per cent of people working in the creative and performing arts sector will lose their jobs. In contrast, she notes the generous bailout packages offered to the arts by Australia's international counterparts:

> In the UK, a relief fund will provide GB£162 million … The German government has provided a €50 billion package … The US government has released US$75 million … In contrast, the Australian government has pledged just an additional AUD$27 million to support the sector … Most Australian artists and arts workers will not benefit from the current measures.
>
> *(Caust, 2020)*

There is not scope in this essay to address the deep damage currently being inflicted on the Australian arts economy under COVID. Here we focus primarily on community making resulting from digital performance. However, as the contrast between funding support packages among various countries makes plain, 'the loss to our country may be greater than just economic' should the arts sector fail to recover (Caust, 2020). This loss raises concerns that can be theorised through the work of Lupton (2019) on digital health, as well as Whiting (2019) and Whiting and Carter's (2016) research into arts and music access as a public good. Lupton works with Jane Bennett's vital materialism to analyse the agency that health apps have in creating a more-than-human assemblage of health. She says:

> Human-app health assemblages generate a range of relational connections, affective forces and agential capacities, responding to and working with the affordances of the technologies and the fleshy affordances of human bodies … highlighting the ways in which apps offer opportunities for people to enact identities and embodiments, make forceful connections and to affect and be affected.
>
> *(Lupton, 2019: 136–137)*

Lupton's positioning of the human in conjunction with technology as a measure of health shows us how Isol-AID could be considered a route towards creating community wellbeing through live-streamed performance. Whiting and Carter (2016) write about the live music scene in Australia in relation to access. They argue that access to the arts is broadly considered a 'public good' and that lack of access is a limitation in equality: 'In Australia, access tends to be equated with policies and initiatives enabling performers and audiences with a disability to participate in the arts and music sectors' (Whiting and Carter, 2016: 1). However, Whiting (2019) later writes that 'music is the catalyst for participation, but it is the social aspect of a performance that helps to maintain the scene's vibrancy' (Whiting, 2019: 56). We agree that having access to the arts and the social aspects of music scenes and arts communities is vital to achieving certain social determinants of health and wellbeing. Instagram Live can be considered a good way of providing these health benefits amid socially distant times, a new mode of digital community health.

Rhiannon was sent an Instagram message from an Isol-AID fan, saying that as someone who is chronically ill and often unable to attend live gigs, this completely digital festival has been a long-anticipated event:

> I know isolation is a new thing for many, but as someone with a chronic illness (who mostly doesn't have access to mainstream festivals) I didn't realise I had been waiting years to have something like this enter my life … It gave me a sense of hope that moving forward this could be something that disabled and able people of all access can work on doing together moving forward.

This points to the fact that many live music festivals across Australia have limited access for people with disabilities. Considering options such as live streaming at festivals in the future could open up music communities to a more diverse audience, and while the COVID crisis continues would broaden the discussion around accessibility to the arts in general (Qi and Hu, 2020). An article from Sunrise Medical, a leading innovator in mobility research and mobility product design, states that music festivals are often hosted on grassy areas, which present limited options for those who need mobility aids, as 'mosh and enclosure areas do not provide seating space for attendees, which means that seated wheelchair users can be disadvantaged, even endangered, by a predominantly standing and overly enthusiastic crowd' (Sunrise Medical, 2020). The writer also notes that 'fortunately, our society is moving towards a more inclusive future and is beginning to understand how important accessible entertainment events are, which means that disability-friendly music festival attendance options are on their way' (Sunrise Medical, 2020). Examples of such events include *Ability Fest, Sounds & Vibes*, and *Feel the Beat*, among others.

Petra Kuppers, a disability culture activist, artist and scholar, has examined the importance of accessibility to live performance and theatre. Her book *Theatre and Disability* (Kuppers, 2017) examines the conceptual, sensory and creative engagement that theatre performed by people with a disability generates through the frameworks of disability as spectacle, narrative, and experience. Similar points are also advanced in the research of Michele Decottignies (2016). Describing the findings of a national survey concerning Canadian disability arts, Decottignies (2016) suggests that we should not see access to the arts as disabled people gaining access to mainstream arts, but should reshape the ways the arts are made through disability as a form of cultural autonomy. Through her work with the Restless Dance company, Anna Hickey-Moody also considers the agency of disability as it is generated through affirmative narratives of disability as ability. Hickey-Moody (2009: 61) frames this production of agency through affect and dance:

> As an affirmative realm, integrated dance theatre produces [+−bodies] in a performance ensemble. It materially changes the ways bodies with intellectual disability are known and is expressive of change within social imaginaries. It shifts the understandings of viewing bodies by staging new relationships between dancers and audience members … Bodies are no longer intellectually disabled, or not intellectually disabled.

Access needs to be seen not as a matter of able-bodied people 'giving' access to those who are disabled, but a rethinking of what it means to perform live in and of itself. As we are reminded through the limitations of the pandemic, accessibility is not just a disability issue, it is also an issue for those who are rural, regional, or isolated in other ways. Rhiannon discusses the concept of bridging live digitally broadcast performances and live physical audiences together in the future, something many artists are experimenting with amid COVID:

> I imagine there could be a potential where at your show, the same way that you would record through the mixing desk, there can be a camera set up at the back of the venue that ties in with the sound engineer so the live video and sound could be streamed at the same time. With something like that, the venue could take a percentage as well. So, say you sell out The Corner Hotel for 800 tickets, and then you sell another 1,000 online, that's more revenue for the venue, and then there's less pressure for the audience to be spending money at the bar, or even to make it into the show if they can't, kind of thing … it's inclusive of those people who can't physically make it to venues, whether it's physically unable through a disability of some kind, or they live too far away. At the end of the day, you as an artist can still perform live at that venue, because I agree, there is nothing like a live performance in a venue, but it's the fact that there's no choice for people who physically can't get there, they just don't get to see their artists. Whereas all you have to do is, the same way you hire an engineer to give your audience in the front of the stage good sound, you can hire an engineer to give the same to, yeah, people watching on a screen.

Live streaming in tandem with live performance at venues might be one useful way to bridge gaps between accessibility to the arts and creative expression as a public health benefit. Another consideration we would like to see occur is a revision of government support payments. Acknowledging the nature of the already unstable gig economy in Australia, Rhiannon recommends:

> I think that JobKeeper[2] would be good if there was a section that was specifically for the arts community, just being able to navigate an average of like, what would you have made this month on average if you had kept those gigs? But it just isn't really made that simple through JobKeeper or JobSeeker. So, yeah, that would help, if there was something more curated around the arts community. It's just a blank form right now that's not really suited to our needs.

Rhiannon's response highlights a broader community sentiment which shows the current lack of support and governmental recognition artists are receiving in Australia. Our colleagues at RMIT University, Shelley Brunt and Kat Nelligan (2020), released a report on the media narratives which surround the Australian music industry and mental health due to COVID. Their commentary reveals grave concerns for music industry workers and artists alike, as they are considered 'low on the [government's] list of priorities' (Chief Medical Officer Brendan Murphy, quoted in Brunt and Nelligan, 2020), when ironically, in a public health crisis, this is when we need them the most.

Conclusion

In the COVID pandemic, live streaming has been a key means through which artists have continued to connect with their audiences/community and audience members have been able to access live art and music. Our posthumanist understanding of community calls for a more nuanced account of accessibility to the arts that features digital live streaming as a robust and vitally important method of community making. Access to art is an essential part of community health and wellbeing; innovative methods of connection such as Isol-AID have never been more needed for those of whom, due to disability or (social) distance, are limited from accessing physical venues. Social policy in Australia needs to draw on the social prescribing literature to show how the social determinants of health can be mediated through creativity and artistic expression. The agency of technology, art and music – things which serve as mediators in the posthuman community assemblage – need to be considered against a backdrop of public health and community cohesion.

We argue for a number of changes:

1. A revised government support system which takes into account the precarity of arts employment in Australia.
2. A community of audience members and venues which embraces live streaming as a method of live performance and who economically and culturally support digitally broadcast gigs and shows.
3. A revision of the way in which the arts is valued in Australia that considers the greater health implications of access to the arts.

We acknowledge the consequences of expecting artists to continue to perform live online during huge funding and job losses; as such, Australians need to find a suitable way to support artists to continue to create their work throughout crises. A more targeted approach from policy makers, social services and funding bodies, which acknowledges artists for the work they do in building community both on- and offline, is necessary. Cultural policy would benefit from looking to the Isol-AID creators as an example of how to provide access to the arts in a time where hope is waning. It is in finding this balance, embracing this in-betweenness of live-streamed shows through a screen and as performed through the fleshy humanness of in-person gigs, where we see the potential sustainment of the arts sector in Australia. There is much we can learn from artists and the ways they make community through more-than-human assemblages amid difficult times. In the case of Isol-AID, this togetherness is facilitated by digital technology, reminding us that community is, and always has been, posthuman.

Notes

1 We base our understanding of wellbeing on that of the World Health Organization, which states that 'wellbeing is a keyword in the WHO definition of health: a state of complete physical, mental and social wellbeing and not merely the absence of disease or infirmity' (World Health Organization, 2020).
2 JobKeeper and JobSeeker are some of the available governmental social support schemes in Australia that offer fortnightly payments to those who are unemployed or seeking work.

References

Auslander P (2008) *Liveness: Performance in a Mediatized Culture* (2nd edition). New York: Routledge.

Barber S and Naepi S (2020) Sociology in a crisis: Covid-19 and the colonial politics of knowledge production in Aotearoa New Zealand. *Journal of Sociology* 56 (4): 693–703.

Barker S (ed.) (2019). *Mental Wellbeing and Psychology: The Role of Art and History in Self Discovery and Creation*. London: Routledge.

Bennett A and Rogers I (2016) *Popular Music Scenes and Cultural Memory*. Basingstoke: Palgrave Macmillan.

Bhatia M (2020) COVID-19 and BAME Group in the United Kingdom. *The International Journal of Community and Social Development*, 2 (2): 269–272.

Braidotti R (2013) *The Posthuman*. Cambridge: Polity Press.

Braidotti R (2019) *Posthuman Knowledge*. Cambridge: Polity Press.

Brunt S and Nelligan K (2020) The Australian music industry's mental health crisis: media narratives during the coronavirus pandemic. *Media International Australia*. Epub ahead of print.

Caust J (2019) The continuing saga around arts funding and the cultural wars in Australia. *International Journal of Cultural Policy* 25 (6): 765–779.

Caust J (2020) Coronavirus: 3 in 4 Australians employed in the creative and performing arts could lose their jobs. *The Conversation*, 20 April. Retrieved from https://theconversation.com/coronavirus-3-in-4-australians-employed-in-the-creative-and-performing-arts-could-lose-their-jobs-136505 (accessed 8 October 2020).

Camic PM and Chatterjee HJ (2013) Museums and art galleries as partners for public health interventions. *Perspectives in Public Health* 133 (1): 66–71.

Chen MY (2012) *Animacies: Biopolitics, Racial Mattering, and Queer Affect*. Durham, NC: Duke University Press.

Decottignies M (2016) Disability arts and equity in Canada. *Canadian Theatre Review* 165 (January): 43–47.

Diamond E, Varney D and Amich C (eds) (2017) *Performance, Feminism and Affect in Neoliberal Times*. New York: Palgrave.

Fleming E and Whitaker J (2019) The art of public health and the wisdom of play. In: Tonkin A and Whitaker J (eds) *Play and Playfulness for Public Health and Wellbeing*. London: Routledge, pp. 50–64.

Fuchs C (2020) Everyday life and everyday communication in coronavirus capitalism. *tripleC* 18 (1): 375–399.

Fullagar S and Pavlidis A (2020) Thinking through the disruptive effects and affects of the coronavirus with feminist new materialism. *Leisure Sciences*. Epub ahead of print.

Harris A and Holman Jones S (2016) *Writing for Performance*. Rotterdam: Brill/Sense Publishers.

Harris A and Holman Jones S (2019) *The Queer Life of Things*. London: Routledge.

Hickey-Moody AC (2009) *Unimaginable Bodies: Intellectual Disability, Performance and Becomings*. Leiden: Brill Sense.

Kimberlee R (2015) What is social prescribing? *Advances in Social Sciences Research Journal* 2 (1): 102–110.

Kuppers P (2017) *Theatre and Disability*. Basingstoke: Palgrave Macmillan.

Lupton D (2019) The thing-power of the human-app health assemblage: thinking with vital materialism. *Social Theory & Health* 17 (2): 125–139.

Mastandrea S, Fagioli S and & Biasi V (2019) Art and psychological wellbeing: linking the brain to the aesthetic emotion. *Frontiers in Psychology* 10. Retrieved from www.frontiersin.org/articles/10.3389/fpsyg.2019.00739/full (accessed 11 January 2021).

Morgan G and Nelligan P (2018) *The Creativity Hoax: Precarious Work in the Gig Economy*. New York: Anthem Press.

Nikolic M and Skinner S (2019) Community. *Philosophy Today* 63 (4): 887–901.

Phelan P (2004) *Unmarked: The Politics of Performance* (5th edition). New York: Routledge.

Qi F and Hu L (2020) Including people with disability in the COVID-19 outbreak emergency preparedness and response in China. *Disability & Society* 35 (5): 848–853.

Richterich A (2020) When open source design is vital: critical making of DIY healthcare equipment during the COVID-19 pandemic. *Health Sociology Review* 29 (2): 158–167.

Robinson L, Schulz J, Khilnani A, Ono H, Cotten SR, Mcclain N, Levine L, Chen W, Huang G, Casilli AA and Tubaro P (2020) Digital inequalities in time of pandemic: COVID-19 exposure risk profiles and new forms of vulnerability. *First Monday* 25 (7). Retrieved from https://journals.uic.edu/ojs/index.php/fm/article/view/10845 (accessed 8 October 2020).

Rogers N (1993) *The Creative Connection: Expressive Arts as Healing*. Mountain View, CA: Science and Behaviour Books.

Sunrise Medical (2020) Accessibility at music festivals. Retrieved fromwww.sunrisemedical.com.au/blog/accessibility-at-music-festivals (accessed 8 October 2020).

Stickley T and Hui A (2012) Social prescribing through arts on prescription in a UK city: participants' perspectives (part 1). *Public Health* 126 (7): 574–579.

Stickley T and Duncan K (2007) Art in Mind: implementation of a community arts initiative to promote mental health. *Journal of Public Mental Health* 6 (4): 24–32.

Straw W (1991) Systems of articulation, logics of change: communities and scenes in popular music. *Cultural Studies* 5 (3): 368–388.

Stuckey HL and Nobel J (2010) The connection between art, healing, and public health: a review of current literature. *American Journal of Public Health* 100 (2): 254–263.

Taylor S and Luckman S (2020) New pathways into creative work? In: Taylor S and Luckman S (eds) *Pathways into Creative Working Lives*. Basingstoke: Palgrave Macmillan, pp. 267–281.

Whiting S (2019) 'You're not strangers if you like the same band': small venues, music scenes, and the live music ecology. PhD thesis, RMIT Research Repository, RMIT, Melbourne.

Whiting S and Carter D (2016) Access, place and Australian live music. *M/C Journal* 19 (3). Retrieved from https://journal.media-culture.org.au/index.php/mcjournal/article/view/1085 (accessed 8 October 2020).

Whiteley S (2012) Counterculture: music theory, and scenes. *Volume! La Revue des Musiques Populaires* 9 (1): 6–16.

World Health Organization (2020) Social determinants of health. Retrieved from www.who.int/teams/social-determinants-of-health#:~:text=Media%20centre-,About%20social%20determinants%20of%20health,global%2C%20national%20and%20local%20levels (accessed 8 October 2020).

PART IV

Healthcare practices and systems

11

STRANGE TIMES IN IRELAND

Death and the meaning of loss under COVID-19

Jo Murphy-Lawless

A brother's farewell

A man is standing on a bench close to a window of a hospital. One of the people who has died in the hospital from COVID-19 is the brother of the man looking in the window. The man has dragged the bench over to the window to take his last glimpse of his brother. There will be no wake, no open coffin, no gentle stroking of the dead man's hands in affection and farewell, no large funeral Mass, no gathering of tea, whiskey and sandwiches, as are the traditions in Ireland.

In Ireland, our not-too-distant history of famine, epidemic death and loss form the cultural backdrop to our funeral traditions, which have continued despite our glossy internationalised economy, the latter a tangible result of neoliberal 'time-space compression' (Harvey, 1989). During the initial lockdown in Ireland, from March 2020, our funeral traditions were no longer open to us and, like the man in the photograph, we had to rely on makeshift farewells. Our world had collapsed inward.

The winter influenza crisis in neoliberal Ireland

The World Health Organization's (WHO) report about significant numbers of pneumonia-like cases in Wuhan appeared on New Year's Eve 2019; a time when the focus of public concern in Ireland was the annual winter outbreak of influenza and its management by our ramshackle health services. Irish hospitals were enmeshed in the winter flu crisis: people on trolleys in jammed emergency departments a principal measurement of how badly our health services perform.

The current configuration of Ireland's health services reflects a history grounded in the state's indifference to those who cannot pay for healthcare. Its exclusionary and means-tested basis has consistently restricted the public structures of, and access to, both general practitioner (GP) services and hospital care, while protecting private medicine (Murray, 2006; Burke, 2009a). Political arguments about health inequalities and the pressing social obligation that treatment should be on the basis of need have been left hanging for many decades. During the 'Celtic Tiger' years from 1990 to 2007, when unemployment melted away, macroeconomic indicators indicated outstanding growth, and government budget surpluses kept growing (Donavan and Murphy, 2013: 16), our healthcare system remained unreformed, except for centralising administration in a costly and controversial new body called the Health Services Executive (HSE).

The neoliberal thesis that private healthcare is more efficient and takes pressure off public services was openly encouraged by a political establishment that pursued this direction vigorously for over two decades, with the twin focus of establishing private hospitals and a deregulated private health insurance market to open up 'competition'. This inequitable system was rightly termed 'Irish apartheid' (Burke, 2009a), leading to poorer health outcomes for people unable to pay for private medicine and subject to ever-lengthening public waiting lists (Wall, 2017; Edwards, 2018); for example, public patients have faced significant delays with respect to initial cancer diagnoses, 25 times longer than for private patients (Cullen, 2016).

Such consequences, while most onerous for patients consigned to the public waiting lists regardless of their individual levels of pain or disease progression, also impacted on clinicians in training, non-consultant hospital doctors dealing with those public lists and nurses, midwives and other healthcare professionals, all of whom faced overwhelming challenges in trying to provide satisfactory care in the public system. At the time the first cases of COVID were announced by WHO, the Irish state had one of the most unequal systems of healthcare in the EU: the unworkable private/public mix resulted in 'unequal experiences and outcomes for different sections of the population benefiting those with more money over those with less' (Burke, 2009b). Ballooning state expenditure on health; damaging healthcare scandals with legal payouts running to hundreds of millions; plummeting workforce numbers; qualified healthcare staff affected by burnout and lack of opportunities emigrating; too great a reliance on foreign doctors and nurses who were arguably needed in their own countries; the first nurses' and midwives' strike in 20 years: all these elements and more constituted the unreformed mess the country faced in January 2020 (Staines, 2017; Cullen, 2019a, 2019b, 2019c, 2020a; Wall, 2019).

On 2 January 2020, the HSE published figures about hospital admissions for the winter seasonal flu outbreak: 1,373 admissions, with 45 patients in intensive care. There had already been 22 flu-related deaths during this outbreak. The HSE stated that although hospital throughput was improving, the severity of the flu outbreak had placed huge pressures on overstretched resources, leaving 404 patients waiting on trolleys that morning to be admitted to wards. HSE officials calculated that the flu season would last another five weeks (Cullen, 2020b). There was detailed national news coverage and families were urged to send in photographs and accounts of the acute overcrowding in emergency departments to news outlets. Ambulance drivers issued a bulletin stating that without reforms their service was 'running on empty' (Cullen, 2020c). That same sense of exhaustion, frustration and being stretched far beyond personal capacity could have been elicited from all frontline healthcare workers and worried families endeavouring to support very sick relatives.

On 14 January, a general election was called. Our broken health service was a major issue confronting politicians in press conferences and media interviews during the campaign, with total health waiting lists numbering 677,000 people, of which more than 100,000 were waiting more than 18 months for a scheduled appointment or treatment (Horgan-Jones and Wall, 2020). The population of Ireland is 4.92 million people. The election over and votes counted, no single party could form a coalition, so Ireland had only an acting government when the coronavirus finally arrived.

The strange times of COVID

Distant rumbles of COVID were met at the end of January 2020 with broad assurances from HSE public health doctors that the health services were 'fully prepared' and would be able to deal with any cases that might arrive but that the 'likelihood' remained low (Cullen 2020d). Getting through the end of the winter flu epidemic remained the major concern at HSE press briefings. As a signed-up performer to globalised world production, Ireland is dependent for its supply chains on a growing trade with China, but we had no direct passenger traffic to Wuhan. The WHO described the virus as SARS-like; we had just one case of the SARS virus in 2003 (Cullen, 2020e). The initial understanding then was that with no direct links to Wuhan and assuming this virus behaved like SARS, Ireland's health services could manage because we were a low risk.

The contradictions between local place (often perceived as 'stable') and the flexible space/s of globalisation, with the urgent need for capital accumulation processes to overcome the former by the latter so as to ensure continuing expansion, make 'time-space compression' inevitable (Harvey, 1989). Even as we tried to understand a SARS-like virus as a very minor threat compared with our annual flu epidemic, we were plunging into what David Harvey describes as an 'overwhelming sense of *compression* of our spatial and temporal worlds' (Harvey, 1989: 240; emphasis in the original). Our radio programmes began to carry interviews with Irish people living in Wuhan and their stories of being locked in, of food shortages and the tedium of being restricted to online communication were shaping a new vocabulary for us. The WHO announcement that the spread of the virus constituted a public health emergency 'of international concern' was followed the next day (31 January 2020) by the first diagnosed case in Italy.

While we waited through February, barely knowing for what, matters were accelerating for our medical professionals. The reality of our health services forcibly confronted them. As more information emerged about the nature and speed of the coronavirus transmission, they were working to do the impossible. No reconfiguration within our hospitals and health services has happened without months, years and decades of wrangling between professional, managerial and political interest groups. With respect to the now certain arrival of COVID, suddenly the shouting stopped. Hospitals swiftly reworked physical layouts and procedures for infection control and tried to tackle the outsize issues of staff shortages, shortages of intensive care beds and the associated shortages of resources and equipment (Coyne, 2020; Mitchell, 2020). Clinicians gained as much information as possible.

An emigrant country by history, in the contemporary globalised world Irish people are more often at the top of the 'emergent hierarchy of mobility' (Bauman, 1998: 88) as skilled professionals. Using their professional networks, clinicians asked their colleagues, first in China and then in Italy, what were the most urgent priorities. We had one of the lowest intensive bed capacities in EU countries: 5.2 per 100,000 of the population compared with the European average of 11.5 per 100,000. An Italian doctor posted the following warning: 'You will not recognise or prepare fast enough for the sudden influx of critically-ill patients and they will keep coming' (quoted in Mitchell, 2020).

On 29 February 2020, our first case was confirmed: someone who had travelled back from northern Italy. The less familiar images of Wuhan and its empty streets were replaced in our media by images from Italy inexplicably collapsing under the weight of the pandemic. On the same day, the first COVID death occurred in Ireland. Collectively we could not breathe. On 12 March, at a hastily arranged early morning press conference, our Taoiseach (prime minister) addressed the country about the initial lockdown measures the government was imposing, including the immediate closure of schools and universities. He told us: 'I know that I am asking people to make enormous sacrifices. We're doing it for each other … Acting together, as one nation, we can save many lives' (Irish Government News Service 2020).

Within days, shops and workplaces closed. Festivities for St Patrick's Day on 17 March, ordinarily held in every town and drawing hundreds of thousands of tourists from abroad, were cancelled. The Taoiseach made a second national address on St Patrick's Day in which he outlined further severe curtailment measures, reinforcing the public health language about COVID, the social codes of behaviour necessary to bring down virus transmission and the new mechanisms set in place to oversee this national emergency. He reminded us that the upsweep of cases 'is making big demands of our healthcare staff, big demands of every single one of us' and again drew on the theme of acting together in calling for a critical national effort. His plea for social solidarity was premised on the national importance of St Patrick's Day:

> This is a Saint Patrick's Day like no other. A day that none of us will ever forget. Today's children will tell their own children and grandchildren about the national holiday in 2020 that had no parades or parties but instead saw everyone staying at home to protect each other.
>
> *(Department of the Taoiseach 2020)*

It was a shrewd speech, employing a touchstone of Irishness to invoke the sense of *patria* of which Joseph Dunne writes, that despite the 'sheer historical contingency' of being Irish, 'what matters to me, what I care about, what brings me joy or sadness, are … bound up with this country' (Dunne, 2002: 72). The government invoked this sensibility again when the HSE launched a recruitment drive on St Patrick's Day. The Irish Medical Organisation reported on national news that evening that 25 Irish doctors in Perth, Australia, had resigned from their jobs on the morning of St Patrick's Day and booked flights home immediately. When they qualified, many had not been offered jobs in our hospitals or left Ireland because working conditions were so poor. They knew the realities which no government would admit publicly, that the 'modern, vibrant economy and society' Ireland chooses to portray on the international scene, 'safely distanced' from its darker past (Kirby, Gibbons and Cronin, 2002:7), remains connected to that past in ways far less publicly acknowledged than St Patrick's Day: in this instance by the abject failure to care for its people by building a reliable healthcare system open to all. Yet Irish-born healthcare professionals were coming home to be here for people who would need their skills.

After St Patrick's Day, case numbers escalated, the airports were closed to all but emergency flights, and the skies were as empty as the streets and roads beneath. We were in the strangeness of COVID times.

Loss in COVID times

Emigration is long woven into the fabric of Ireland. During the Great Famine of 1845–1852, it is estimated that one million people left the country. Emigration continued throughout the 20th century (Ó Gráda, 1997: 212–217) and into current times following the most recent economic crash. Halfway through COVID lockdown, the historian Diarmaid Ferriter wrote of how the Irish emigrant must hold simultaneously the worlds of 'dislocation and integration' which becomes acutely difficult when a family member is dying at home (Ferriter, 2020).

COVID made us all emigrants of sorts: those who were unable to travel back and those of us still in Ireland who were unable to be present with family members who were dying. With a handful of exceptions, hospitals and nursing homes closed their doors to relatives. Nursing and medical staff, masked and gowned, did their best to link dying patients and their relatives via speakerphones and iPads, but the loss was compounded with the deep pain of not being there: 'This plague robs you of moments you can't comprehend. Stroking her hair when she is sick. Holding her hand when she is dying' (quoted in Kenny, 2020). Pádraig Byrne, whose brother Francis died in hospital, spoke poignantly of his experience on national radio of saying goodbye at a distance (as shown in Figure 11.1): 'It did comfort me, I felt I was there. It was the only way I could say my last goodbye to him' (quoted in Pollak, 2020a).

The importance in Irish culture of being physically present in times of death long predates the nationalist Catholic period of the late 19th and early 20th centuries. German travellers to Ireland before the Great Famine, fascinated by the depth of poverty and the fact 'that the one political system contains the richest country in the

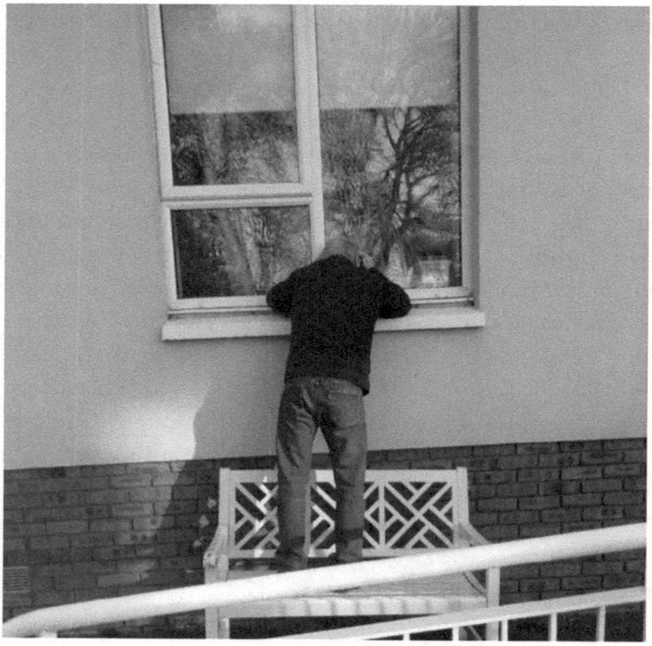

FIGURE 11.1 Pádraig Byrne looks through the hospital window at his brother Francis, who died from COVID-19

Source: Felicia Byrne/RTÉ Liveline

world and one of the poorest' (Bourke, 2011: 7), found themselves taken with the emotion and distinctive care shown in how Irish people responded to death:

> Lately I rode to Carrick-on-Suir, and when I was approaching the town I came upon a funeral … It was a genuinely ancient Irish burial, with wailers of the kind that are to be seen in these times.
>
> *(Karl Gottlob Küttner, 1783 and 1784, quoted in Bourke, 2011: 42)*

In an account of the wake and funeral of a young woman from a poor family in county Limerick in 1832, an anonymous German traveller describes going to the family's cottage with the son of the landlord with whom he is staying. The young woman, clad in a white shroud with long white ribbons, is laid out on a bedstead, three candles alight 'on the best candlesticks that could be borrowed from various neighbours'. The tiny house is packed with dozens of people. The following day the funeral takes place with young boys dressed in white leading the procession, followed by 'six old women in scarlet capes' who 'raised their voices … in an ancient Irish keening … The bereaved father and mother … followed directly behind the coffin led by friends, after which there came a procession of about fifty persons' (Anonymous I, 1832, quoted in Bourke, 2011: 170–177).

Throughout the history of poverty, emigration and the Famine itself – during which a million people died – the Irish have learned much about grief, loss and the sheer localness of memories about death (Tóibín, 2004: 19–23). An understanding of place to publicly express the importance of death and the depth of loss is something we have not entirely traded away. To borrow from David Lloyd (2003: 220), we are able to decide not to 'lose our loss in order to become [the] good subjects of modernity'. Lloyd argues that the period of the Famine marks 'the historical emergence of a new kind of Irish subject … who embodies a peculiar weave of memory, damage and modernity' (Lloyd, 2003: 206). As a society, we have used that weave in these COVID times, creatively, urgently, in seeking concrete expression for the strong insistent need to publicly mark loss and death.

Official information on the conduct of funerals was issued at the outset of the COVID outbreak in Ireland. Public funerals ceased regardless of cause of death. Numbers attending were limited to 10 people, strictly physically distanced. Double body bags had to be used for those who had died from COVID and open coffins were ruled out. The country was forced to make immediate adjustments. For example, early on in the pandemic, a small parish in west Kerry, Baile an Fheirtéaraigh, unable to hold either wake or funeral Mass under COVID restrictions, did what they could. To honour the woman who had died and to support her family, the community lined the two-kilometre distance on either side of the road from the church to the graveyard: 'Death and wakes are so central to community life here in west Kerry and people were frustrated that this pandemic was preventing them to pay their respects to a wonderful woman and her family' (Mac an tSíthigh, 2020).

It was hard. Here is one man's account of his mother's funeral in a large Dublin church:

> It was a very desolate affair, made worse by the dreaded social distancing. Looking around, you would be forgiven for thinking we were all strangers and that Margaret wasn't loved. It isn't fair. We've attended Margaret's funeral but it doesn't feel like we've been able to grieve properly.
>
> *(Quoted in Kenny, 2020)*

In June, the national broadcaster RTÉ screened two television programmes which had documented the experiences of staff and patients in St James Hospital, Dublin, one of the state's largest hospitals, during the height of the pandemic. St James lost 79 patients to COVID (Power, 2020). One of the people to die was a 97-year-old man, Patrick Commins, who had been supported in sheltered housing by his care worker. After Patrick died, the care worker brought in a suit for him to be dressed in, along with his treasured pocket-watch to be put into his hands. She is filmed singing his favourite song to him one last time before nurses prepare to put his body into the double body bag. As they work, the nurses talk gently to Patrick as if he is not dead (Power, 2020).

In his excoriating critique of modernity, Bauman (1994: 4–5) argues that its lethal division of the 'regular, predictable, and controllable from the contingent, erratic, unpredictable and going out of hand' has the consequence of a moral code, a rules-based morality which teaches people to hear 'only the voice of reason'. It is precisely that version of modernity, where feeling is subordinated to reason, which Lloyd argues does not quite fit with Irish society. No matter how modern and global we declare ourselves, we are 'a culture which is constantly athwart … modernity' (Lloyd, 2003: 216), not least in how we respond to the human problem of loss. As the pandemic moves away from its initial peak, the question is whether Ireland from its position of being 'athwart' can evolve different understandings of what it might need and want in a post-COVID world.

Ní neart go cur le chéile

Every townland in Ireland has a GAA club, the Gaelic Athletic Association, which promotes the Irish sports of hurling, Gaelic football and camogie. There are 2,200 clubs across the island. As soon as lockdown measures were announced, the clubs began to distribute leaflets offering help to people needing practical support. These leaflets often bore the Irish saying *Ní neart go cur le chéile* ('There is no strength without unity').

This sense of the word 'community' was mobilised and reinforced at many such levels across Ireland, as we moved towards the other totemic day in the official Irish calendar, Easter Sunday, the anniversary of the Easter Rising in 1916. This day commemorates Irish nationalists publishing the Proclamation of Independence that declared Ireland a sovereign republic and took up arms in rebellion against the British state, paving the way for the War of Independence 1919–1921, and ending in the creation of the Irish Free State in 1922. The annual public commemorations for 1916 were cancelled. Instead, President Michael D Higgins issued a message speaking of the pandemic's impact 'as we strive together to come to terms with the Coronavirus and its consequences' for 'our Irish family' including 'the Irish community abroad … a community united by its roots to Ireland, but also by these shared values that our Irishness embodies'. He urged every Irish home 'to place a light in their window … a time so important in the symbolism of our Irish Independence', a light to underscore 'our shared solidarity' (President of Ireland's Office, 2020).

However, Ireland, the enthusiastic adopter of neoliberal economics, now faced consequences. We were confronting multiple contradictions about 'social solidarity' and what we might hope to designate as a 'community' in this global crisis. Always a stratified society, Ireland has been further riven by how we have engaged in the current globalised world. We have steep inequalities of income, 'one of the most market unequal countries in the EU' (Sweeney, 2020: 20). Since the economic collapse of 2008 and the austerity which followed, Ireland has faced a housing and homelessness crisis of devastating proportions, which the pandemic made still more acute. If the public health directive to the 'community' to limit the spread of COVID was to 'stay at home', many thousands of people trapped in precarious rented housing, emergency accommodation, direct provision for asylum-seekers, or none at all, had to face the lack of housing security when it was vital to avoid transmission (Hearne, 2020).

Ireland has the third-highest number of foreign-trained doctors of all OECD countries (Pollak, 2020b); many of our nurses are also foreign-trained (Cullen, 2019c). The HSE hired 2,500 new staff during the crisis, yet Irish-born staff who have returned from abroad are unsure they will have anything other than short-term contracts (Hutton, 2020). Worst of all, the wholesale privatisation of residential social care and the growth of private nursing homes with poor state regulation over the last two decades led to the disaster of 1,030 COVID deaths in 167 care facilities; almost all deaths were people who were elderly and infirm, representing 62 per cent of the state's total number of COVID deaths (Horgan-Jones and Carswell, 2020).

Turning aside, living 'athwart'

By the end of July 2020, Ireland had recorded 26,077 confirmed cases of COVID and 1,763 people had died. Amazingly, despite our health services bearing the hallmarks of the ill-paid 'highly gendered, racialized and ethnicized' frontline of this vicious neoliberal global economy (Harvey, 2020), there were only eight healthcare worker deaths recorded.

President Higgins stated in his Easter address that 'this crisis, too, will pass but its severity and magnitude are, to a large extent, in our own hands' (President of Ireland's Office, 2020). There is an inference here that acting once as we should and must enables us to act again. In the early stages of the pandemic, rather than the repeated organisational sabotage of our healthcare system (Burke, 2009b), we acted to give a chance to nurses, doctors and healthcare workers to do their work. It was far from perfect, as high rates of COVID infection among nurses indicate (Irish Nurses and Midwives Organisation, 2020). Nonetheless we stepped apart from the canon of neoliberal thought, its ruthless profit-taking, and remembered bonds, about loss and death, and staff in our health system were finally enabled to accomplish what was 'self-evident' all along, caring for people on the basis of need alone. Thus, we may have come to recognise the urgency to change our system permanently. Perhaps Ireland will now seek to implement, as a matter of urgency, the 2018 all-party reform plan called Sláintecare in order to achieve universal healthcare (O'Connor, 2020).

A scene in the *RTÉ Investigates* television documentary on St James Hospital brings this need to change the Irish healthcare system emphatically home, when a nurse speaks after the camera has shown her zipping up a double body bag. She tells us it is 'an awful thing to hear … it's the last thing you hear when you close your eyes at night' (Power, 2020). We have heard that nurse and have begun to understand how we need to be, as a society, for her. We have finally understood the uses of how we deal with grief, why lining the roads to the graveyard connects with a time when people, in readying their potatoes for planting, 'kibbed their spuds on the one day' (kibbing is the back-breaking labour of digging the holes for the potato seed in stony, unforgiving soil) before the 'cold individualism' of the current economic order encroached (Mac Suibhne, 2017: 98).

The capacity to care for people who need extensive care, including caring for our health workers, is a form of 'commonage' (Mac Suibhne, 2017: 98), a 'training' for the very solidarity that will 'cut against the individualising strategies of neoliberalism' (May, 2012: 133). Learning to carry this through in a post-pandemic Ireland will determine our capacity to turn aside from the worst excesses of globalised modernity. We can oppose its 'ubiquitous and seemingly endless violence' by 'producing and reproducing a life that lies athwart' (Lloyd, 2003: 217), a life that valorises how we care. The pandemic has jolted us into remembering, from where we have been, from our sense of localness and place, that we know how to resist. In another Irish saying often repeated during these months, which teaches us what caring embodies in and about our society, 'We live in the shadow of each other' – *Ar scáth a chéile a mhaireas na daoine.*

References

Bauman Z (1994) *Alone Again: Ethics after Certainty*. London: Demos.

Bauman Z (1998) *Globalization: The Human Consequences*. Cambridge: Polity Press.

Bourke E (2011) *'Poor Green Erin': German Travel Writers' Narratives on Ireland from Before the 1798 Rising to After the Great Famine*. Frankfurt am Main: Peter Lang.

Burke S (2009a) *Irish Apartheid: Healthcare Inequality in Ireland*. Dublin: New Island.

Burke S (2009b) Apartheid nature of our health system must end. *Irish Times*, 27 July. Retrieved from www.irishtimes.com/opinion/apartheid-nature-of-our-health-system-must-end-1.793197 (accessed 28 May 2020).

Coyne E (2020) Hospital team protected patients by prepping for Covid-19 in January. *Irish Independent*, 26 June. Available at www.independent.ie/irish-news/hospital-team-protected-patients-by-prepping-for-covid-19-in-january-39317517.html (accessed 5 July 2020).

Cullen P (2016) Public patients wait up to 25 times longer for cancer tests. *Irish Times*, 26 April. Retrieved from www.irishtimes.com/news/health/public-patients-wait-up-to-25-times-longer-for-cancer-tests-1.2624303 (accessed 24 August 2020).

Cullen P (2019a) Medical-negligence cases set to cost record €374 million next year. *Irish Times*, 19 November. Retrieved from www.irishtimes.com/news/health/medical-negligence-cases-set-to-cost-record-374-million-next-year-1.4088074 (accessed 24 August 2020).

Cullen P (2019b) Reliance of Ireland's health system on overseas doctors has risen to record levels. *Irish Times*, 2 October. Retrieved from www.irishtimes.com/news/health/reliance-of-ireland-s-health-system-on-overseas-doctors-has-risen-to-record-levels-1.4038004 (accessed 30 May 2020).

Cullen P (2019c) Ireland's reliance on nurses coming from abroad rises further. *Irish Times*, 18 April. Retrieved from www.irishtimes.com/news/health/ireland-s-reliance-on-nurses-coming-from-abroad-rises-further-1.3863770 (accessed 30 May 2020).

Cullen P (2020a) Emigration of medical staff blamed on wide range of problems. *Irish Times*, 6 February. Retrieved from www.irishtimes.com/news/health/emigration-of-medical-staff-blamed-on-wide-range-of-problems-1.4163081 (accessed 30 May 2020).

Cullen P (2020b) Number of flu deaths hits 22, but outbreak 'may have peaked'. *Irish Times*, 2 January. Retrieved from www.irishtimes.com/news/health/number-of-flu-deaths-hits-22-but-outbreak-may-have-peaked-1.4129014 (accessed 1 June 2020).

Cullen P (2020c) First week of 2020 'worst ever' for hospital overcrowding. *Irish Times*, 10 January. Retrieved from www.irishtimes.com/news/health/first-week-of-2020-worst-ever-for-hospital-overcrowding-1.4135852 (accessed 1 June 2020).

Cullen P (2020d) HSE says it is ready to deal with new coronavirus from China. *Irish Times*, 23 January. Retrieved from www.irishtimes.com/news/health/hse-says-it-is-ready-to-deal-with-new-coronavirus-from-china-1.4149430 (accessed 2 June 2020).

Cullen P (2020e) New Coronavirus is increasingly likely to spread to EU, health bodies warn. *Irish Times*, 23 January. Retrieved from www.irishtimes.com/news/health/new-coronavirus-is-increasingly-likely-to-spread-to-eu-health-bodies-warn-1.4148375 (accessed 2 June 2020).

Department of the Taoiseach (2020) National address by the Taoiseach, St Patrick's Day. 17 March. Retrieved from www.gov.ie/en/speech/72f0d9-national-address-by-the-taoiseach-st-patricks-day (accessed 29 June 2020).

Donavan D and Murphy A (2013) *The Fall of the Celtic Tiger: Ireland & the Euro Debt Crisis*. Oxford: Oxford University Press.

Dunne J (2002) Citizenship and education: a crisis of the Republic? In: Kirby P, Gibbons L and Cronin M (eds) *Reinventing Ireland: Culture, Society and the Global Economy*, pp. 69–88. London: Pluto Press.

Edwards E (2018) Waiting times for healthcare in Ireland 'amongst worst in Europe'. *Irish Times*, 29 January. Retrieved from www.irishtimes.com/news/health/waiting-times-for-healthcare-in-ireland-among-worst-in-europe-1.3372624 (accessed 25 August 2020).

Ferriter D (2020) When going back can be as difficult as staying. *Irish Times*, 16 April. Retrieved from www.irishtimes.com/opinion/diarmaid-ferriter-when-going-back-can-be-as-difficult-as-staying-1.4253589 (accessed 10 June 2020).

Harvey D (1989) *The Condition of Postmodernity: An Enquiry into the Origins of Cultural Change*. Cambridge, MA: Blackwell.

Harvey D (2020) Anti-capitalist politics in the time of COVID-19. *Jacobin*, 20 March. Retrieved from https://jacobinmag.com/2020/03/david-harvey-coronavirus-political-economy-disruptions (accessed 4 July 2020).

Hearne R (2020) Covid-19 shows we need a new housing direction in Ireland. *Irish Examiner*, 3 June. Retrieved from www.irishexaminer.com/opinion/commentanalysis/arid-31002971.html (accessed 5 July 2020).

Horgan-Jones J and Wall M (2020) More than 677,000 on hospital waiting lists last month, new figures show. *Irish Times*, 14 February. Retrieved from www.irishtimes.com/news/ireland/irish-news/more-than-677-000-on-hospital-waiting-lists-last-month-new-figures-show-1.4174195 (accessed 1 June 2020).

Horgan-Jones J and Carswell S (2020) The human cost of Covid-19: Ireland's care homes with the most deaths revealed. *Irish Times*, 28 May. Retrieved from www.irishtimes.com/news/ireland/irish-news/the-human-cost-of-covid-19-ireland-s-care-homes-with-the-most-deaths-revealed-1.4264170 (accessed 10 June 2020).

Hutton B (2020) Doctors returning to fight Covid-19 feel betrayed, says IMO. *Irish Times*, 19 June. Retrieved from www.irishtimes.com/news/health/doctors-returning-to-fight-covid-19-feel-betrayed-says-imo-1.4283771 (accessed 29 June 2020).

Irish Government News Service (2020) Statement by An Taoiseach Leo Varadkar on measures to tackle Covid-19 Washington. 12 March. Retrieved from https://merrionstreet.ie/en/News-Room/News/Statement_by_An_Taoiseach_Leo_Varadkar_On_measures_to_tackle_Covid-19_Washington_12_March_2020.html (accessed 29 June 2020).

Irish Nurses and Midwives Organisation (2020) 88% of healthcare workers with COVID got virus at work. Press release, 12 June. Retrieved from www.inmo.ie/Home/Index/217/13594 (accessed 15 June 2020).

Kenny C (2020) Grief in a pandemic: 'Not being able to see him in his final hours was heartbreaking'. *Irish Times*, 18 April. Retrieved from www.irishtimes.com/life-and-style/people/grief-in-a-pandemic-not-being-able-to-see-him-in-his-final-hours-was-heartbreaking-1.4230528 (accessed 30 June 2020).

Kirby P, Gibbons L and Cronin M (2002) Introduction: The reinvention of Ireland a critical perspective. In: Kirby P, Gibbons L and Cronin M (eds) *Reinventing Ireland: Culture, Society and the Global Economy*. London: Pluto Press.

Lloyd D (2003) The memory of hunger. In: Eng D and Kazanjian D (eds) *Loss: The Politics of Mourning*, pp. 205–228. Berkeley, CA: University of California Press.

Mac an tSíthigh S (2020) Kerry community finds way to pay respect to parishioner amid restrictions. 20 March. Retrieved from www.rte.ie/news/coronavirus/2020/0320/1124388-funeral-kerry/ (accessed 20 March 2020).

Mac Suibhne B (2017) *The End of Outrage: Post-Famine Adjustment in Rural Ireland*. Oxford: Oxford University Press.

May T (2012) *Friendship in an Age of Economics: Resisting the Forces of Neoliberalism*. Lanham, MD: Lexington Books.

Mitchell S (2020) Leading the charge against COVID-19. *Business Post*, 15 March. Retrieved from www.businesspost.ie/health/leading-the-charge-against-covid-19-c2061fa7?auth=registered (accessed 20 March 2020).

Murray P (2006) The evolution of Irish health policy: a sociological analysis. In: Cluskey D (ed.) *Health Policy and Practice in Ireland*. Dublin: UCD Press.

O'Connor A (2020) Sláintecare more relevant in post-Covid-19 world than ever before. *Irish Times*, 14 April. Retrieved from www.irishtimes.com/opinion/sl%C3%A1intecare-more-relevant-in-post-covid-19-world-than-ever-before-1.4227857 (accessed 1 June 2020).

Ó Gráda C (1997) *A Rocky Road: The Irish Economy since the 1920s*. Manchester: Manchester University Press.

Pollak S (2020a) Coronavirus: Dubliner recalls poignant farewell to brother. *Irish Times*, 8 April. Retrieved from www.irishtimes.com/news/social-affairs/coronavirus-dubliner-recalls-poignant-farewell-to-brother-1.4224400 (accessed 9 April 2020).

Pollak S (2020b) Thousands of nurses and doctors from abroad form backbone of our Covid-19 battle. *Irish Times*, 20 May. Retrieved from www.irishtimes.com/news/health/coronavirus-heroes-ireland-has-looked-after-us-so-it-s-time-to-return-the-favour-1.4257305 (accessed 1 June 2020).

Power E (2020) Inside Ireland's Covid battle. *Irish Times*, 29 June. Retrieved from www.irishtimes.com/culture/tv-radio-web/inside-ireland-s-covid-battle-you-might-be-fighting-tears-before-the-first-ad-break-1.4292043 (accessed 6 July 2020).

President of Ireland's Office (2020) Message to the Irish at home and abroad at Easter 2020. 10 April. Retrieved from https://president.ie/en/media-library/news-releases/message-to-the-irish-at-home-and-abroad-at-easter-2020 (accessed 29 June 2020).

Staines A (2017) Irish healthcare can be fixed if we find the moral courage. *Irish Times*, 20 May. Retrieved from www.irishtimes.com/opinion/irish-healthcare-can-be-fixed-if-we-find-the-moral-courage-1.3089333 (accessed 1 June 2020).

Sweeney R (2020) *The state we are in: inequality in Ireland 2020*. Dublin: FEPS, TASC.

TóibínC (2004) The Irish Famine. In: TóibínC *and* FerriterD (eds) *The Irish Famine: A Documentary*. London: Profile Books, pp. 3–36.

Wall M (2017) Waiting lists in public hospitals 'out of control'. *Irish Times*, 20 July. Retrieved from www.irishtimes.com/news/health/waiting-lists-in-public-hospitals-out-of-control-1.3161240 (accessed 25 August 2020).

Wall M (2019) Health reforms impossible due to workforce crisis, doctors warn. *Irish Times*, 13 August. Retrieved from www.irishtimes.com/news/health/health-reforms-impossible-due-to-workforce-crisis-doctors-warn-1.4052223 (accessed 30 May 2020).

12

BETWEEN AN ETHICS OF CARE AND SCIENTIFIC UNCERTAINTY

Dilemmas of general practitioners in Marseille

Romain Lutaud, Jeremy K. Ward, Gaëtan Gentile and Pierre Verger

Introduction

The emergence of a new deadly virus such as COVID-19 acts as a reminder that uncertainty is a feature of modern societies. In France, as in many other countries, the uncertainty regarding the virus during the early months of the pandemic was coupled with heated public arguments on many aspects of the authorities' handling of the crisis: the best ways to use the limited number of diagnostic tests available, whether the general lockdown was put in place too late, and whether uniform confinement was the correct strategy. These debates stem from the absence of the ideal type of solution usually sought for medical problems: a vaccine or effective medical treatment. It is therefore not surprising that one of the most heated debates to have surfaced in the first stages of the pandemic, was over whether a cure for COVID had been found in the form of the drug hydroxychloroquine. This debate, and the social life of this drug, epitomise the issues pertaining to uncertainty that the medical world faces during epidemic outbreaks.

Hydroxychloroquine became global news in March 2020, when US President Donald Trump publicly touted its efficacy. Since then, debates around this drug have mainly been framed in terms of the decline in trust in science and the spread of fake news. But this sort of framing does not help understand why such a debate can emerge at that particular moment of the epidemic. As with many scientific issues, such as vaccines (Goldenberg, 2016), reducing the debate to a confrontation between science on one side and, on the other, an illiterate public and anti-science actors, tends to overlook the rationality behind people's apparently misguided behaviour. In the case of hydroxychloroquine, this common explanation reducing complex attitudes to degrees of 'scientific literacy' is challenged by the fact that many doctors in developed countries (and in France in particular) prescribed this drug during the early phases of the pandemic (Sermo Report, 2020). How can we explain the fact that so many people with very advanced medical training agreed (at least partly) with the ramblings of Donald Trump? The attitude of practising doctors towards hydroxychloroquine constitutes an ideal site to explore the issues they face in contexts of epidemic outbreaks and the relationship between their practice, scientific research and authorities' recommendations. This is particularly apparent in France, the epicentre of the worldwide debate on hydroxychloroquine.

In France, hydroxychloroquine made the front pages in March 2020 and remained one of the main themes of the media coverage of COVID during the following month-and-a-half. This media sequence was sparked by the publication of a clinical trial purporting to show the spectacular effect of using hydroxychloroquine in combination with azithromycin (Lemaire and Michel, 2020). This study sparked a worldwide debate – and gave Donald Trump so much hope. It was conducted by a team led by the person who would become the main defender of this drug: Didier Raoult. This infectious disease physician is the director of the Institut Hospitalo-Universitaire Méditerranée Infections (IHU), a public research and treatment facility dedicated to infectious diseases located in Marseille.

The debate touched upon crucial questions relative to how doctors should act in the face of scientific uncertainty: should practising doctors be the ones making the judgement call for their patients, and what degree of certainty must be reached before action should be taken in times of crises? In their defence of the use of hydroxychloroquine, Didier Raoult and other experts put forward their moral obligations as doctors to care for their patient and the cognitively superior knowledge they develop at patients' bedsides. This approach was presented as well tailored to the urgency of crises, as opposed to the unethical and scientifically dubious nature of randomised trials and 'big data'. But do these discourses fit the actual experience of practising physicians? What do practising physicians' attitudes towards hydroxychloroquine tell us about the issues they face in times of epidemic outbreaks and how they manage to solve them?

In this chapter, we shed light on the difficulties faced by French general practitioners (GPs) confronted by the outbreak of COVID and the resources at their disposal to solve them. We will focus in particular on how they solved the question of whether to prescribe hydroxychloroquine. Drawing on the sociology of the relationship of general practice with uncertainty, we show what kinds of problems this prescription was believed to solve. This assists in understanding the limits to the persuasive power of official guidelines and GPs' resistance to evidence-based medicine. Our argument constitutes a first attempt at bringing together the results of a wider research project involving the analysis of 32 interviews; two surveys conducted among 142 GPs in Marseille and 1200 GPs in France respectively; messages exchanged on Whatsapp local GP group and mailing lists; an analysis of the coverage of the hydroxychloroquine debate in the French national press; and three surveys conducted among representative samples of the French population. It will also draw on Romain Lutaud's experience of working as a general practitioner in Marseille during the COVID pandemic.

'Professional prudentialism'

In recent years, French sociologists have taken a great interest in how general practitioners deal with the prevalence of uncertainty in their daily practice, arguing that this is a key element of general practice. There are a number of reasons for this: two different diseases can be difficult to distinguish because their sets of symptoms are very similar; symptoms appear differently from one person to the other; the boundary between being healthy and being sick is often blurry; and recommending a treatment implies taking into consideration the medical idiosyncrasies of each individual as well as their psychological and socioeconomic situation (Bloy, 2008; Jutel and Nettleton, 2011). Furthermore, GPs are aware of the limits of their own knowledge (Bloy, 2008; Fox, 1988).

GPs' professional ethos reflects the prevalence of uncertainty and the imperative to take into consideration a great diversity of potentially contradictory factors (Dodier, 2007; Löwy, 2007). French sociologist Florent Champy has coined the term 'professional prudentialism' to describe this type of professional ethos also found among architects (Champy, 2018). Because doctors, just like architects, are faced with problems that are too complex to be solved by the mechanistic application of abstract rules, their practice is characterised by a form of practical wisdom:

> Practical wisdom is the approach required for acting in specific and complex situations, which produce a high level of uncertainty. It is also the virtue required for protecting others (whether clients of professionals or citizens in the field of politics) from the damage incurred whenever uncertainty is not properly acknowledged. It is the very opposite of a mechanical implementation of rules that are too abstract (that is, devised without any reference to the practical situations to be dealt with), of formalised procedures, of scientific knowledge or of routines. It implies that particular attention is to be paid to the concrete aspects of the situation, to its singularity and complexity.
>
> *(Champy, 2018: 83)*

GPs' particular form of professional prudentialism (or practical wisdom) emphasises the importance of interaction with patients as well as the past experience of doctors in their practice (Bloy, 2010; Dodier, 2007). Thinking about GPs' practice in terms of this professional ethos rather than in terms of the extent of their medical knowledge sheds light on a number of important phenomena, such as the liberty doctors can take with official recommendations and some of the resistance faced by evidence-based-medicine in the medical world (Champy, 2018; Dodier, 2007; Löwy, 2007; Urfalino et al., 2002). Indeed, 'professional prudentialism' entails a certain distance towards all sources of information: each one can only be just one of many elements taken into consideration. Because best practice recommendations can only integrate a very limited number of parameters, they are often seen as unsatisfactory and can easily be seen as contradicted by GPs' past experience (Bloy,

2010; Champy, 2018; Dodier, 2007). This strand of research helps shed light on a number of aspects of GPs' experience of the COVID epidemic.

The uncertainties of an emerging disease

To understand French GPs' practices during the first months of the epidemic, we must first understand the uncertainties brought about by COVID. The first type of uncertainty relates to COVID's clinical expression, which did not facilitate a doctor's diagnostic process: the disease may or may not manifest itself as fever, coughing, angina or asthenia. All these signs are inconsistently found during the consultation and are not specific to COVID. Also, clinical knowledge about the disease was evolving as new atypical symptoms were reported, either in published studies or feedback that circulated on social networks (for instance, isolated diarrhoea, vascular acro-syndromes, anosmia). In addition, each symptom may have a different prognostic value for the disease and therefore lead to different ways of organising patient follow-up.

The second type of uncertainty relates to the biological tests for SARS-CoV-2 (by nasal swab). These tests did not initially produce diagnoses of certainty for two reasons. The first reason was that, in the first phase of the pandemic, access to the coronavirus test in France was restricted. Apart from severe cases in hospital, the only people eligible for the test were symptomatic people at risk of complications, or health professionals. General practitioners were therefore unable to confirm the diagnosis for their patients if they were asymptomatic, just as they could not offer a test to symptomatic patients without pre-existing health conditions. The second reason was the lack of reliability of the nasal test, which at first had an estimated sensitivity of 56–83 per cent. As a result, many French physicians continued to consider their patient as possibly having COVID despite a negative test.

It must be said that, in France, GPs were not left completely alone to decide what to do. They received recommendations from a number of different actors, including the French Ministry of Health and French regional health agencies (ARS). The French national college of teaching general practitioners quickly set up a website (coronaclic.fr) summarising the various recommendations and care management algorithms. However, the desire to avoid confronting GPs with so much uncertainty transpired through the initial official pathway of care for patients potentially affected by COVID, which in the first month, meant that GPs were bypassed. When displaying symptoms associated with COVID, people were supposed to call a dedicated number that prompted them either to contact the hospital emergency system in case of serious illness or to organise a teleconsultation with their GP. Two reasons for this particular organisation were put forward: the lack of validated treatment; and the risk of viral contamination in waiting rooms in doctors' offices.

But, as with many other recommendations, this official pathway did not solve many of the issues faced by GPs in France. Many GPs we interviewed felt that abandoning the usual organisation of care pathways (with GPs on the front line as gatekeepers) in the name of the exceptional nature of the crisis was unjustified and irrelevant, especially because of the break in their relationship with the confined patient it created. This was not the only problematic recommendation. In our survey study conducted among 1200 French GPs, we also found that only half the respondents considered official recommendations regarding COVID to be sufficient or applicable, and two-thirds felt that they changed too often (Lutaud et al., 2020a). In late April (after the peak of the epidemic), French health authorities, under pressure from general practitioners' representatives (learned societies and unions), gradually put GPs back on the front line of the system.

GPs' views on the hospital-centred strategy, as well as the gap between official recommendations and what GPs perceived to be the reality of their daily work with COVID, must also be interpreted against the backdrop of a general context of a complicated relationship between the medical profession and the health authorities in France for more than two decades. Indeed, the multiplication of health scandals around purported or documented episodes mishandled by public health agencies, as well as GPs' exclusion from the management of various epidemics over the past few decades, has undermined medical professionals' trust in health authorities (Mullard, 2011).

What is evident, therefore, is that the official recommendations on how to deal with COVID did not solve the problems faced by a number of GPs. The case of COVID also illustrates why GPs are often dissatisfied by official guidelines which can only integrate a very limited number of parameters (Champy, 2018). This phenomenon is particularly exacerbated in France, because patients' pathway of care is very centred on the relationship with one independent GP working mostly alone, rather than with medical collectives (Bloy, 2008; Rosman, 2010). In the case of COVID, GPs' tendency to consider official recommendation as just one of the many resources at their disposal seems to have been exacerbated by a distrust of public health authorities. The relationship between doctors' attitude towards uncertainty – their professional prudentialism, trust in public health authorities and the uncertainties specific to this particular epidemic – were made particularly visible around the issue of the prescription of hydroxychloroquine.

The problem with hydroxychloroquine

To understand how hydroxychloroquine found its way onto the list of uncertainties faced by GPs, it is necessary to reconstitute the unfolding of public debates. On 25 February 2020, Didier Raoult published a video on YouTube, in which he downplays the seriousness of the virus and touts the efficacy of hydroxychloroquine both as a treatment and as a prophylactic (Lemaire and Michel, 2020). This video was followed by some very cautious discussion in the national media of the possible merit but also the great uncertainties of using this drug. Expert voices mainly focused on the necessity to wait for clinical trials proving that the treatment was indeed effective and safe. But the debate really caught on after the publication at the end of March of a study conducted by Didier Raoult and his colleagues purporting to show the effectiveness of hydroxychloroquine when taken in combination with an antibiotic (Azithromycin) as soon as the symptoms appear.

The publication was followed by interviews with Didier Raoult as well as segments dedicated to criticism of the study's methodology: small number of patients, irregularities in the inclusion of patients, selection biases, publication in a journal in which one of the authors acts as an editor. One of the main arguments put forward was the fact that most people infected by SARS-CoV-2 develop only mild symptoms and the claim that the use of hydroxychloroquine was likely to cause cardiac problems in at-risk patients. Defenders of the drug claimed, on the contrary, that it was well known, that it was very rarely associated with such side effects and that the low risk could easily be made even lower by performing electrocardiograms before and after treatment. Criticism was voiced by prominent scientists, including members of the scientific advisory board on COVID appointed by the president (Lemaire and Michel, 2020).

The use of hydroxychloroquine was defended not only by Raoult, but also by other prominent professors of medicine as well as some politicians. Ten days after the publication of this first study, the Haut Conseil de la Santé Publique (HCSP), one of France's most prominent sources of expertise on medical matters, recommended using it only for very severe cases and the Académie de Médecine and the Académie des Sciences voiced their concern at the use of pharmaceuticals without having scientifically evaluated them first. This led the government to publish new decrees authorising this treatment only in hospitals and for severe cases (25 and 27 March). Didier Raoult and his colleagues later published two other studies with bigger sample sizes, but they were also severely criticised for their methodology and weakness of their results (Lemaire and Michel, 2020). For GPs, these developments meant that until the end of March they were free to prescribe hydroxychloroquine in any context. The decree published on 26 March explicitly placed boundaries around GPs' medical judgement. It stated that the drug could only be used for rheumatoid arthritis and lupus, and for the prevention of actinic dermatitis.

These rapidly changing recommendations did not help avoid the type of issues described in the previous section. From the outset, some doctors perceived recommendations as not allowing any guidance in the field and as an infringement of their freedom of prescription (Foucart and Vincent, 2020). Indeed, we found in our interviews that a number of doctors had very different judgements from those of the health authorities about the dangers of hydroxychloroquine, in particular because many of them had previous experience of prescribing it. Finally, it is important to note that one of the difficulties faced by GPs on this particular issue was patients' demand for treatment. The great publicity given to hydroxychloroquine meant that patients themselves often tried to weigh in on the decision being made by GPs about prescribing this treatment. Several surveys conducted between April and May showed that between 35 and 60 per cent of the public believed in the efficacy of this drug against COVID (Coconel Report, 2020). This popular opinion was reflected in our survey among 1200 GPs: 27 per cent reported that the controversy over hydroxychloroquine had made it difficult for them to deal with patients' treatment requests. This proportion was even higher in the areas most strongly affected by the epidemic and those closest to Marseille (Lutaud et al., 2020a).

The case of hydroxychloroquine illustrates one particular issue faced by best practice recommendations in contexts such as the early phases of the COVID outbreak. Because little is known about the novel coronavirus and possible treatment, much of their content pertains to how doctors should deal with uncertainty. On an issue such as hydroxychloroquine, official recommendations can be boiled down to a general reaffirmation of some of the norms at the core of evidence-based medicine, including the fact that doctors should recommend a treatment only if there is a demonstrated effect documented by published research. But these principles have been the object of much resistance within the medical community, especially among GPs in France, because they run counter to the classical professional identity and ethos of GPs presented in the previous section, which entails that best-practice recommendations can only be source of information informing practice. French sociologists have documented the many liberties taken by GPs with best practice recommendations (Urfalino et al., 2002). But more importantly, this strand of research has shown that some of the standard ways of dealing with this uncertainty may contradict best practice recommendations. During COVID, these resources have often played in favour of hydroxychloroquine use, as we will now see.

How GPs solved their dilemmas

Confronted with the uncertainties of the initial phases of the COVID outbreak, GPs resorted to four main pathways to resolving their problems:

- a restrictive logic;
- testing therapeutic solutions;
- division of labour; and
- the patient-centred care approach.

A restrictive logic

The first pathway favoured compliance with official recommendations, and this is consistent with the idea that official recommendations are meant to help doctors solve the problem of uncertainty. Most doctors have followed the national recommendations regarding COVID in general and hydroxychloroquine in particular: even if, as noted in the previous sections, many had issues with them or perceived them to be lacking in many areas. This 'restrictive logic' is best described by Rosman: 'drug prescribing becomes a practice practiced with reserve or parsimony' and in line with recommendations for good practice (Rosman, 2010: 23). But interestingly, compliance with official recommendations was often presented as the product of coordination with other GPs (often via local professional networks) rather than as resulting directly from consulting official documents. However, many of GPs' other standard modes of resolution of uncertainty could run counter to these official recommendations.

Testing therapeutic solutions

One particular problem with best practice recommendations is that most of the time they presuppose a strict separation between the diagnosis and the treatment. However, this does not take into consideration the fact that GPs routinely use treatments as diagnostic tools and/or see the stabilisation of the patient's situation as the priority before committing to a diagnosis (Urfalino et al., 2002). This latter aspect is particularly important, given that the short-term improvement of their health is often a priority for patients and is therefore an expected outcome of the consultation. In the case of COVID, we saw a significant proportion of doctors trying out various treatments. A survey conducted among 470 doctors found that around 20 per cent have prescribed a drug outside of its marketing authorisation and that 70 per cent of the time the treatment had been hydroxychloroquine (Medscape Report, 2020). In our interviews with GPs, they described prescribing other aetiological treatments, mainly antibacterial drugs such as macrolides and cephalosporins, despite evidence of a bacterial superinfection.

This way of conceiving pharmacological treatment corresponds to Rosman's (2010) logic of 'instant repair' through drugs. Indeed, a number of constraints beyond knowledge and uncertainty bear on the doctor–patient interaction: the need to establish and maintain the relationship with the patient; the need for legitimacy; and the management of the consultation in a context where patients expect a quick improvement of their situation. In this context, providing patients with a prescription often constitutes a solution to a complicated problem. International comparisons of prescription practices suggest that using drugs as a tool to respond to the patient's complaint seems to be particularly popular among French GPs (Rosman, 2010).

Division of labour

Another standard resource of GPs when dealing with uncertainty is the referral to specialists (Champy 2018) This practice recognises the limit of the GPs' capacity to handle uncertainty. It is therefore a resource that runs counter to their ethos of 'professional prudentialism', which explains why there is often a reluctance to refer to a specialist or to a general hospital. This reticence grounded in the idea that these healthcare providers will not take into consideration the patient as a whole (Bloy, 2010; Champy, 2018).

In the case of COVID, this strategy played in favour of hydroxychloroquine use in the epicentre of the controversy, Marseille. The specificity of the city was to offer two competing options to GPs. One of the assets of the IHU in Marseille was its ability to perform as many COVID diagnostic tests as necessary. This meant that, in a context where the availability of tests was rare and where many tests performed were unreliable, the IHU provided a solution to these problems for GPs. However, when coming to the IHU, patients would be offered treatment with hydroxychloroquine. For doctors who were convinced by the arguments in favour of hydroxychloroquine, delegation of the patient's care was therefore a very satisfying solution. For doctors who were still undecided on the subject, it could also appear as an acceptable solution because they trusted that doctors at the IHU would make an informed judgment on whether treatment was warranted and would follow their patients satisfactorily (being specialists of infectious diseases). But for GPs who did not believe in hydroxychloroquine, the fact that the IHU provided such a crucial service meant that they had to balance not testing against the possible risks of hydroxychloroquine and their patients' ability to refuse it. In our interviews, several such doctors described this exact situation and their decision to refer their patient to the IHU. But more importantly, many told us that their patients went straight to the IHU without consulting them first, because they wanted to be tested.

The patient-centred care approach

Finally, the main way of coping with the uncertainties surrounding COVID was via discussions with patients. Physicians increasingly face patients who make specific requests or even demands for treatment, based on their own search for information and on non-medical considerations. This reflects the process of empowerment (Lupton, 1995), through which patients have strengthened their willingness and ability to take effective care of themselves and their health. In response to, or in parallel with, patient empowerment, GPs in particular have developed patient-centred care, defined as 'care that is respectful of and responsive to individual patient preferences, needs, and values' and that ensures 'that patient values guide all clinical decisions' (Barry and Edgman-Levitan, 2012). Overall, we found that most general practitioners sought to 'normalise' care with their patients by relying on the professional values traditionally attached to family medicine: to accompany, reassure, be at their patients' side in this anxiety-ridden period, and support them in their decisions.

Medical consultations can be encounters where forms of lay and expert knowledge meet. On controversial or highly uncertain objects such as in the case of COVID and as already observed in our work on chronic Lyme disease, which focused on the recognition of the patient's diagnostic activity, the patient's perspective is reinforced (Lutaud et al., 2020b). This was particularly striking when it came to the issue of hydroxychloroquine. We found that whether patients asked for this treatment or not bore significantly on the unfolding of the consultation and, more importantly on whether the doctor would prescribe it. This was especially striking for GPs in Marseille. Our interviews suggest that patient demand for testing and hydroxychloroquine was one of the major determinants of whether the GPs sent their patients to the IHU.

Conclusion

In this chapter, we have sought to explain and better understand why some French GPs recommended hydroxychloroquine by applying a sociological lens. By identifying doctors' practices during COVID, we hope to have shown the limits of explaining attitudes that different from the scientific consensus by a lack of knowledge or understanding. The study of medical work is therefore helpful to understand attitudes and behaviours that deviate from the scientific norms in general, including those of the lay public. Focusing on the practices of general practitioners in the context of the healthcare system in France shows that a different form of explanation exists: a more sociological one (see, for instance: Pescosolido, 1992; Urfalino et al., 2002) that puts scientific knowledge in the context of the practices in which they are mobilised and the problems people try to solve. Indeed, GPs' work entails drawing on the type of knowledge published in academic journals and compiled to formulate best-practice recommendations. But it also relies on other types of knowledge, such as past experience, knowledge of the situation of the patient and knowledge arising within the interaction with the patient. This is even more the case in contexts in which new infectious diseases have emerged, such as COVID, where academic medical knowledge was initially scarce.

An insightful analysis of GPs' work practices implies going beyond comparing their behaviour and beliefs with what official recommendations say, and interpreting discrepancies and compliances as reflecting different levels of scientific literacy. It implies understanding GPs' work as a complex problem-solving practice that goes beyond the mechanistic application of knowledge. We believe this is also the case for the public. Explaining why so many members of the French public believed in the efficacy of hydroxychloroquine entails moving away from 'deficit model explanations' to understand how this belief makes sense in the particular context of each person's experience of COVID and the problems they face.

While our focus was on the factors that enabled hydroxychloroquine to be prescribed, we do not want to suggest that all French GPs were in favour of it or that the factors we put forward played in exactly the same way in the practices of every GP. Sociologists have shown that there are a variety of ways of responding to uncertainty among French GPs, characterised by varying degrees of distance towards best practice recommendations (Bloy, 2008). There are various ways of incarnating the 'professional prudentialism' in medicine and differences in how much GPs rely on their practical wisdom rather than on official guidelines (Champy, 2018).

At this stage of our research, we have not been able to identify the precise phenomena leading some GPs to endorse hydroxychloroquine as a treatment, others to suspend their judgement and the rest to reject it. But this initial exploration suggests that patients play a crucial role in this process, which leads us to our final point. In the absence of an effective drug, we have seen, at least in some instances, a form of horizontalisation of knowledge, with some physicians sharing their uncertainties and powerlessness with their patients. In France, as a result of the recent process of institutionalisation of general practice as a 'proper' specialty within the French university system, general medicine has put forward two fundamental principles: the will to integrate the patient in the decision-making process (patient-centred care approach), and to rely on robust knowledge (evidence-based medicine). The COVID crisis has uncovered the potential conflicts between these two principles.

Acknowledgements

Romain Lutaud and Jeremy K. Ward are the co-first-authors of this chapter, for which they contributed equally.

We would like to thank the following: the entire team of the department of general practice at Aix-Marseille university for their broad support throughout this research. Our Family Medicine residents Marie Poirey, Alienor Denoix, Marie Pierre, Manon Mermier and Marie Duez for their involvement in field work and the quality of their interviews. Dimitri Scronias and Gwenaelle Maradan from the ORS PACA, CPTS Actes Santé and its energising leader Jessica Lavigne, the ARS PACA and the URPS-ML PACA in particular Dr Brieussel, and the DRESS (Ministry of Health). Finally, we would like to warmly thank the general practitioners who have given their time in the midst of a health crisis to be by the side of their patients.

References

Barry MJ and Edgman-Levitan S (2012) *Shared Decision Making: The Pinnacle of Patient-centered Care.* Waltham, MA: Massachusetts Medical Society.

Bloy G (2008) L'incertitude en médecine générale: sources, formes et accommodements possibles. *Sciences Sociales et Santé* 26 (1): 67–91.

Bloy G (2010) La constitution paradoxale d'un groupe professionnel. In: Bloy G and Schwever F-X (eds) *Singuliers Généralistes.* Métiers Santé Social. Rennes: Presses de l'EHESP, pp. 21–40.

Champy F (2018) The sociology of prudential activities: from collective commitment to social innovations. *Sociologia, Problemas e Práticas* 88: 79–94.

Coconel Report (2020) Coconel – Note de synthèse no 3. Confinement, masques, chloroquine, vaccin: ce qu'en pensent les Français | ORS Paca. Retrieved from www.orspaca.org/notes-strategiques/coconel-note-de-synth%C3%A8se-n%C2%B0-3-confinement-masques-chloroquine-vaccin-ce-qu%E2%80%99en (accessed 10 October 2020).

Dodier N (2007) *Les Mutations Politiques du Monde Médical: L'objectivité des Spécialistes et L'autonomie des Patients.* Paris: Presses Universitaires de France.

Foucart S and Vincent F (2020) Coronavirus: les généralistes, première ligne invisible face au Covid-19. *Le Monde*, 2 April. Retrieved from www.lemonde.fr/planete/article/2020/04/02/les-generalistes-premiere-ligne-invisible-face-au-covid-19_6035286_3244.html (accessed 10 October 2020).

Fox RC (1988) *L'incertitude Médicale.* Paris: L'Harmattan.

Goldenberg MJ (2016) Public misunderstanding of science? Reframing the problem of vaccine hesitancy. *Perspectives on Science* 24 (5): 552–581.

Jutel A and Nettleton S (2011) Towards a sociology of diagnosis: reflections and opportunities. *Social Science & Medicine* 73 (6): 793–800.

Lemaire F and Michel P (2020) Chloroquine: une saga médiatique. Retrieved from www.acrimed.org/Chloroquine-une-saga-mediatique (accessed 10 October 2020).

Löwy I (2007) Les mutations politiques du monde médical: l'objectivité des spécialistes et l'autonomie des patients. In: Tournay V (ed.) *La Gouvernance des Innovations Médicales.* Paris: Presses Universitaires de France, pp. 303–324.

Lupton D (1995) *The Imperative of Health: Public Health and the Regulated Body.* Thousand Oaks, CA: Sage Publications.

Lutaud R, Scronias D, Ward J and Verger P (2020a) The hydroxychloroquine debate: a therapeutic dilemma for general practitioners. Retrieved from https://deepblue.lib.umich.edu/handle/2027.42/156030 (accessed 10 October 2020).

Lutaud R, Verger P, Peretti-Watel P and Eldin C (2020b) Diagnostic pathways of patients consulting at the infectious diseases ward for presumed Lyme disease: a qualitative descriptive study. Retrieved from https://hal-amu.archives-ouvertes.fr/hal-02915010 (accessed 10 October 2020).

Medscape Report (2020) Impact de la crise du Covid sur l'éthique médicale : résultats d'enquête. Retrieved from https://francais.medscape.com/diaporama/33000220?nlid=136148_2541&src=WNL_mdplscardionews_200629_MSCPEDIT_FR&uac=243754DK&faf=1 (accessed 10 October 2020).

Mullard A (2011) Mediator scandal rocks French medical community. *The Lancet* 377 (9769): 890–892.

Pescosolido BA (1992) Beyond rational choice: the social dynamics of how people seek help. *American Journal of Sociology* 97 (4): 1096–1138.

Rosman S (2010) Les pratiques de prescription des médecins généralistes. une etude sociologique comparative entre la France et les Pays-Bas. In: Bloy G and Schwever F-X (eds) *Singuliers Généralistes*. Métiers Santé Social. Rennes: Presses de l'EHESP, pp. 117–131.

Sermo Report (2020) Largest statistically significant study by 6,200 multi-country physicians on covid-19 uncovers treatment patterns and puts pandemic in context. Retrieved from www.sermo.com/press-releases/largest-statistically-significant-study-by-6200-multi-country-physicians-on-covid-19-uncovers-treatment-patterns-and-puts-pandemic-in-context (accessed 10 October 2020).

Urfalino P, Bonetti E, Bourgeois I and Dalgalarrondo S (2002) *Les Recommandations a L'aune de la Pratique: le Cas de L'asthme et du Dépistage du Cancer du Sein*. Paris: Centre de Sociologie des Organisations.

13

POST-PANDEMIC ROUTES IN THE CONTEXT OF LATIN COUNTRIES

The impact of COVID-19 in Italy and Spain

Anna Sendra, Jordi Farré, Alessandro Lovari and Linda Lombi

Introduction

Italy and Spain endured the early severity of the coronavirus pandemic that some other countries experienced later. At the very beginning, these two countries had two of the highest infection and mortality rates of COVID-19 in Europe, leading to scrutiny of both their health systems and their whole way of life. Starting from a critical analysis of the Italian and Spanish health policies and reforms, the objective of this chapter is to examine how sociocultural factors (intermingled with economy, technology, media and politics) can assist in explaining the impact of COVID in both countries. In the anticipatory phase of the pandemic, the threat of collapse of the health system triggered all the alarms. As the noise increased, the strength of strong and weak ties came into play, combined with a technological and informational saturation of the population. Although this situation was similar in other countries, the Mediterranean idiosyncrasy must be understood 'as a predetermined combination of cultural bias (shared values and beliefs) and specific types of social relationships' (Boholm, 2015: 59). It is in this linkage that cultural dynamics and modes of social interactions coalesce.

Both Italy and Spain responded too little, too late to the governance, management and communication of the pandemic. At first, these countries shared the urgency of adopting severe lockdowns to avoid the collapse of healthcare services, but this limited capacity is not the only way of understanding the impact of COVID in Italy and Spain. Although the issue about whether this decision was made in time will be the subject of ongoing debate, what makes these countries cases worth studying is 'the combination of [...] normatively problematic interactions between social and political context, technological development and citizen behaviour' (Vaccari, 2012: 157). Nevertheless, the first analyses only focused on politics, indicating that the Italian and Spanish responses were based on a mismanaged, unprepared and unexpected policy design (Capano, 2020; Legido-Quigley et al., 2020). This situated both countries at a similar level to the response of the United States and the United Kingdom (Carter and May, 2020; Scambler, 2020), in contrast to other approaches like those of South Korea and Singapore (Lee et al., 2020; Wong and Jensen, 2020).

Historically, it is known which main factors stand in the way of prevention. As Soper (1919) argued in relation to the 1918–19 Spanish influenza pandemic (which despite its name did not originate from Spain), effective prevention must be predicated on three key factors: first, the recognition and appreciation of respiratory infections; second, recognition that the infection is highly communicable and difficult to restrict; and third, how to control it varies depending on the temporality of incubation and the consequences of infection. Although the shadow of the 1918–19 pandemic has been present, the difference 100 years later is that COVID has happened in a different environment (Lovari, 2020). However, as occurred with the 2009 H1N1 pandemic, the balance between preparation and alarmism has again created risks, due to a wicked problem related to the dilemma of under-estimation versus over-estimation:

> Could the legacy of the perceived exaggeration in invoking the 1918 experience as a template for the 2009 pandemic be a loss of trust in future calls for action by public health agencies? Do they risk the fate of the boy who cried 'wolf' too often?
>
> *(Dingwall et al., 2013: 172)*

Identifying the main reasons behind the impact of SARS-CoV-2 in Italy and Spain is complex and may even be unachievable. The overall climate of uncertainty (Rutter et al., 2020), politics and arbitrated measures taken to ensure order and social discipline quickly materialised as a serious lockdown, involving a multitude of physical movement restrictions for the Italian and Spanish populations that challenged these distinctive forms of national identities. A selective analysis of the systemic and informative similarities of this perfect storm allows us to address the analysis from a critical crossroad. Health communication strategies and learning skills are used as threads to interweave the common sociocultural roots of Italy and Spain around trust in politics, media credibility, transparency and accountability. Within this multivariate balance between mistakes and successes, our examination will conclude by pointing out some of the ordinary alterations needed in both countries for integrating the extraordinary consequences of the COVID pandemic.

The best and worst of COVID experiences in Italy and Spain can be evaluated from a common insight of strong similarities. Both countries are proud of the high reputation of their health systems (Miller and Lu, 2018), but also of having two of the longest life expectancies in the world. Further, in terms of attractiveness of location and internal and external mobility of people, both Italy and Spain lead as major tourist destinations. Likewise, both countries share the Latin tendency towards interpersonal physical proximity and the Mediterranean character as signs of a distinctive sociocultural identity. For example, we must not forget that in Italy and Spain, unlike other European countries, physical contact and hugging others is the norm rather than the exception. Therefore, the focus here is not on analysing why the pandemic affected these two countries in such dramatic ways, both in terms of mortality and infection rates. The objective is to delve into how common explanations for the reaction (before, during and after) were based on diffused responsibilities and may be decoded using a fruitful comparative logic, where the individual behaviour and forms of social interaction merges with the collective. In other words, this analysis seeks to demonstrate how the intricacies of reinventing social norms and cultural patterns are all-pervasive (Lapinski and Rimal, 2005).

The burdens of the national health system

Both Italy and Spain introduced a public health system in the late 1970s to middle 1980s (1979 and 1986 respectively) based on principles of: universal and largely tax-financed system; prevalent public funding; decentralisation; and a broad portfolio of services (Petmesidou et al., 2014). During the 1990s, difficulties in managing the health system due to economic sustainability emerged in both countries, as a result of the rise in demand (ageing populations) and the increasing costs of medical technologies. The situation worsened in the following decade, during which both health systems were pressured to cut costs after the global financial crisis of 2008 and the resulting austerity policies taken up by the Italian and Spanish governments. Reforms have taken place in both countries to control pharmaceutical spending, to promote system reorganisation aimed at improving efficiency, or to downsize services covered by public insurance (Serapioni and Hespanha, 2019).

These austerity policies have also had an impact on healthcare personnel, affecting the hiring and career progression of these individuals. Both countries suffer from a shortage of healthcare personnel that has led to an increase in working hours for healthcare professionals, often departing from workforce regulations and causing a consistent burn out of clinical staff (Serapioni, 2018). During the 2000s, both Spain and Italy implemented the process of decentralisation of their health systems through a devolution pathway. These changes led to an increase in the power of the regions (in Italy) and of the autonomous communities (in Spain) in terms of planning, managerial and control responsibilities. The recognition of greater autonomy at the regional level has resulted in significant geographical differences with respect to the quality of care delivery (Aguilar and Bleda, 2016; Pavolini and Vicarelli, 2013). These changes have also hindered the process of digitising healthcare and the integration of information systems, with the consequent difficulty of building electronic databases comprising epidemiological, clinical, organisational and economic data on health and healthcare systems.

Furthermore, a clear shift towards the private management of public healthcare institutions was established in several Spanish regions, which has raised public concern (Aguilar and Bleda, 2016). In Italy, only Lombardy – one of the richest areas in the country – adopted a private-oriented health system (i.e. the so-called 'semi-market' model). Nonetheless, the most recent data showed an increase in out-of-pocket spending by Italian families on healthcare, mainly due to a growing dissatisfaction with the public health services (Giarelli, 2020). Although both countries shared common responses to dealing with the economic crisis, there were also key differences. In the Italian case, legislation promoted greater efficiency in spending, to reinforce the integration in primary care and to ensure the treatment rights. Conversely, the reforms dictated by austerity policies in Spain have started to limit access rights to the Spanish National Health Service (NHS): to the point that many scholars have spoken of a threat to the principle of universality on which the Spanish health system was founded (Serapioni and Hespanha, 2019).

The challenges of responding to COVID in Italy and Spain

Italy and Spain have suffered two of the highest burdens of COVID worldwide. Their capacity to respond to the pandemic has been under tremendous pressure, at least in the most affected areas, where hospitals and intensive care units quickly started to collapse due to the number of severe cases. There have been many cases of infection among health professionals, also due to the lack – at least at an early stage – of personal protective equipment (PPE). Moreover, doctors and nurses who served in the peak of infections and in the most affected areas were overwhelmed by the workload and the emotional impact of the crisis (Arango, 2020; Barello et al., 2020). The governments of both countries have also implemented other measures for sharing public recommendations aimed at reducing the transmissibility of the virus and ensuring the early detection and isolation of individuals with symptoms. However, doing so has proven to be a difficult challenge. In both countries, healthcare decentralisation has resulted in discovering virus cases through criteria defined at the regional level, thus leading to significant geographical differences and difficulties in estimating the total amount of infected people. This situation, in combination with the changes in the process of communicating the mathematical models of COVID to the population, has generated controversies and increased uncertainty (Rhodes and Lancaster, 2020).

At a societal level, measures to control and reduce the coronavirus spread were adopted in both countries, introducing a range of social distancing measures, banning movements between geographical areas, and the closure of schools, universities, museums, restaurants and sporting venues. In this regard, it is essential to consider the sociocultural context of Italy and Spain, especially the role of the elderly. Both Italy and Spain have a demographic structure where older adults (i.e. 65 years or over) represent approximately 20 per cent of the population (around 12 and 9 million respectively) (Eurostat, 2020). The effects of the 2008 financial crisis, including loss of employment, made older people the economic pillars of their families thanks to their retirement pensions (Carrascosa, 2015) and accommodating their younger relatives in their homes. A decade later, almost 20 per cent of Italian and Spanish older adults still live with at least one of their descendants (United Nations, 2019). Additionally, unlike their European counterparts, around 60 per cent of elderly of both countries maintain daily contact with their children (García et al., 2018).

The problem is that older adults have been more affected by responses to the pandemic that seem to be centred on the community rather than the individual, leading to increasing social isolation and psychosocial distress (Rahman and Jahan, 2020). In this context, the ways in which elderly people in Italy and Spain are intimately related with their strong-tie network or living together in nursing homes demonstrate how they are intergenerationally enmeshed in the Latin Catholic religious substrate, not seen as a burden but as a celebrated achievement (Carrascosa, 2015). Indeed, it is undeniable that extended families form part of the identity of Mediterranean cultures, and older adults from this area 'have larger family networks and more social exchange than their counterparts in the non-Mediterranean countries' (Litwin, 2009: 605).

These close connections are also made with friends and acquaintances. Both Italians and Spaniards are highly social citizens with relaxed rules in terms of physical proximity, where leisure practices include reuniting people to have a drink or going out for *tapas*. This way of relating between people could help partially explain the impact of the pandemic in Italy and Spain. Similarly, the sociocultural context surrounding digital transformation and communication may also be implicated in this impact.

The knowledge gaps in terms of technology and information

Both Italy and Spain also share many similarities and trajectories in their transition to digital innovation. Both countries have invested in creating specific legislative frameworks to fully digitise national health systems, often in the context of the e-Health European policies. However, the gap between the assumptions of legislative measures and the speed of the implementation of technological changes, both for public health organisations and citizens, is wide, and has been influenced by financial and technological constraints (Sánchez-García, 2019), along with specific cultural factors. There is an evident discrepancy between the institutional rhetorical discourses and the concrete measures taken to implement digital health policies; mainly due to a general lack of a strategic approach in managing digitisation, the resistance of bureaucracies to organisational changes, and the scarce coordination and integration between central, regional and local levels (Legido-Quigley et al., 2020; Lovari, 2020).

The responsiveness of both countries was impacted by the lack of an efficient integrated information system at the national level. For example, it became evident that lack of technology investments over time has negatively impacted the ability to predict and contain the trend of infection. Notably, there have been significant delays in the production and implementation of a universal mobile app for case self-reporting, as well as apps to support contact-tracing efforts. In Italy, although all citizens could download the official government app (*Immuni*), it was only tested in four regions and by that time the number of new infections had declined significantly. In the case of Spain, different and competitive mobile tools (*STOP COVID19 CAT, AssistenciaCovid19*) were created at the regional level without following a clear national strategy.

Linked to these problems with the efficacy of digital tools is the low level of digital competencies of the Italian and Spanish populations. While organisational complexities have delayed the full implementation of digital health, neither country had extensively invested in digital and health literacy, resulting in a low level of competencies in comparison with other European countries (European Commission, 2017). Disparities between individuals related to their access to online services have limited the flow of effective health communication online, where health-related fake news has proliferated. The arrival of the COVID pandemic, accompanied by a massive infodemic (Pan American Health Organization, 2020), exacerbated the situation of information crises already present in Italy and Spain (Lovari et al., 2021). This was partly expedited by the intense circulation of COVID misinformation on digital media (Salaverría et al., 2020).

Media coverage has also broadened the acceleration of all-pervasive negative consequences in relation to economy, politics and human impacts. The media has been used by politicians and scientists as a battleground for conflicting and contrasting interpretations in association with prophetic opinions and disparate disciplines of expertise. Public discourses focused on symbolic performances or some other forms of populist nationalism addressed to sharing common imageries and collective memories to unity and togetherness (Yabanci, 2020). The existence both in Italy and Spain of right-wing and far-right parties, combined with the decision-making tension between centralised and decentralised authorities, has increased confrontation and contributed to the polarisation of public opinions. Indeed, evidence indicates that COVID led to the dissemination of much political fake news and to a strong politicisation of health-related topics, especially before the lockdown in Italy (Lovari, 2020). This happened, for example, in relation to restrictions, as some politicians used the medical emergency to criticise the government's interventions; with the objective of creating political instability during the acute phase of the pandemic (Ferraresi, 2020; Lovari, 2020).

Similarly, misinformation appears to be linked to conspiracy theories aimed at undermining alliances within the European Union (European External Action Service, 2020). Despite the commitment of digital companies to stop the spread of misinformation, and notwithstanding the strategic partnerships between the World Health Organization and the health ministries, fake news remained difficult to contain for cultural and linguistic reasons as well. Facebook, for example, has not been able to uniformly remove close to 70 per cent of Spanish and Italian-language fake news related to SARS-CoV-2 (Avaaz, 2020).

The impact of epidemics on social relations is also related to different forms of experiential connection via smartphones, tablets and wearable devices, which could generate positive effects on strong- and weak-tie networks (Granovetter, 1973). As Wright (2016: 74) explains, 'social networks tend to be made up of strong ties (such as close friends and family) as well as weak ties (such as co-workers, acquaintances, and people with whom one has infrequent contact)'. In this context, Italy and Spain remain countries with a predominant influence of Catholicism, where solidarity is based on kinship rather than public support from institutions

(Naldini, 2003). This support manifests itself most intensely in times of stress or uncertainty, as in the case of COVID, forcing families to rely once again on the support of their closest networks.

However, the lack of relationship between people living on the same street can also crystalise into a significant tie when health professionals are applauded from the balconies to show solidarity and recognition. This way of sharing emotional support during a disturbing situation of lockdown, with the obligation of staying at home, also involves a latent function of cohesiveness in moments of surprise, uncertainty and fear (Wright, 2016). But this networked society is a reality full of unaccomplished promises, with poor competencies and technological gaps presenting persistent barriers. In addition to political and economic debates about democratic principles, the cultural background and digital inequalities of both countries have limited the success of strategies to deal with an uncertain future.

Compliance with social norms and communication

Confronting the COVID pandemic through human behaviour change involves two complementary fields, health and risk communication, that are gaining recognition for their emphasis on understanding and intervening in communication processes (Rimal and Lapinski, 2009). In particular, three of the most effective recommendations to protect and avoid contagions have been disseminated: washing hands, wearing masks and keeping physical distance. Personal hygiene rests on individual responsibility, whereas the protection with masks involves social interaction patterns where public approval is needed for the sake of duty. Concerning physical distancing, the congruence should be negotiated with the establishment of a code of collective conduct that, for example, would jeopardise ceremonial rituals with crowded meetings (Moore and Burgess, 2011). The challenge here materialises in how these social norms are perceived and integrated into concrete realities of individual and social life and how cultural factors shape the congruence needed to maintain them (Chung and Rimal, 2016).

As Walter et al. (2019: 652) indicate, 'a deeper understanding of normative behaviour should consider social norms as motivational forces that are constructed and reinforced by networks of affiliation'. Masks and hand washing are descriptive norms and their compliance seems easy to understand because their costs could be considered as low in comparison with their effectiveness. Although wearing a mask can be more subject to be negotiated for different reasons (e.g. comfort), hand hygiene depends exclusively on each individual. However, due to the influence of emotions in the perception and evaluation of risks, cultural processes may influence compliance with COVID recommendations (Lupton, 2013). In the context of Mediterranean cultural norms privileging social interactions that tend to be more open, cheerful and supportive than in other European countries, this results in a variability of behaviours within the population; thus adding a layer of complexity to the response strategies of public health authorities. In addition to recent changes in media environments, which have given communication a new role that influences the building of norms (Geber and Hefner, 2019), it is undeniable that social network capital is also a key element of people's attitudes and behaviours (Granovetter, 1973; Wright, 2016).

Post-pandemic world: routes and challenges

There is no doubt that the early months of the COVID pandemic presented a considerable shock to public health, economic and social systems that requires us to plan interventions aimed at preventing similar situations in the future. As the outbreak has dramatically revealed the impact of austerity policies in Spain and Italy of the last decade, there is a clear necessity to increase the resilience of the health system in both countries. This means that it would be necessary to invest substantial resources in healthcare workers, instruments and information systems to reinforce the capacity of these institutions to collect data, detect critical events quickly and disseminate the necessary information across the whole organisation and towards citizenship in an integrated manner. Similarly, the pandemic has highlighted the limits of the reforms on the governance of both health systems. The emphasis on the devolution process has increased geographical disparities and reduced the ability to provide a coordinated response at a national level, and many scholars have urged the need to rethink health systems in a logic of new recentralisation, albeit partial (Giarelli, 2020; Legido-Quigley et al., 2020). This mismanaged regional fragmentation has also challenged the capacity of the system to detect sentinel events and raise public awareness rapidly, despite counting on the support of mobile health apps.

From another perspective, the COVID crisis has pointed out the challenge of reinforcing primary care for preventive intervention. Above all, it is necessary to strengthen the fundamental role of healthcare system gatekeepers, covered by general practitioners, who should have the capacity to provide timely identification of cases to ensure early interventions (Giarelli, 2020). Furthermore, it is also crucial to strengthen the interdependence between healthcare and other systems (e.g. economic, educational, sociocultural), thus promoting a more comprehensive approach to increase the capacity of these institutions to cope with future pandemics. This includes the acceleration of the digitisation processes in Italy and Spain, both from the point of view of infrastructure and services as well as from the perspective of health communication. The severe lockdown restrictions in the early months of the pandemic and the consequent switch to digital forms of communication in Italy and Spain highlighted the disconnect between a rhetoric of digital innovation and the lack of resources to implement digital services and to enhance citizens' online competencies.

The COVID crisis could represent a turning point for digitisation processes and quality of healthcare communication in both countries, especially if parts of the national recovery plans and specific European funds are used for initiating a new route towards digital innovation. This road should be transparent and accountable, but also able to strongly reduce the social and technological inequalities that have characterised

Italy and Spain during the pandemic. It seems that adequate digital skills can empower citizens to access services and information in both ordinary and emergency situations, but it also may lead to the opposite outcome if handled poorly.

In terms of health and risk communication, the COVID crisis has emphasised the lack of specific training in crisis and emergency communication of many public sector organisations, including health institutions. This first social media pandemic has been a major challenge for health communicators; individuals often failed in effectively communicating data and numbers to counteract the infodemic and thus reduce the impact of false narratives. With the increasing diversification of social media platforms, 'individuals' health [...] will be shaped by a multitude of social forces, each of which can mediate different kinds of health contagion processes' (Zhang and Centola, 2019: 104). Mitigating the spread of fake news seems to involve coordinated efforts between authorities, mass media and digital companies, but it also appears crucial to invest in education and digital literacy for developing a critical awareness of the use of digital technologies that could be useful for facing future health crises. In other words, the strengthening of comprehensive population-centred responses lies on finding answers concerning how the mechanisms of public concern will operate to engage in coherent protection rules or in what ways the forms of interaction will change (Zinn, 2008).

Added to all these routes and challenges, the Latin cultural roots of both Spain and Italy have endured in at least in three factors: elderly people, social proximity and cultural values, all mixed within the alteration of everyday routines and collective rituals. Overall, the COVID crisis has been a stress test for the health system, politics, economy and sociocultural seams. What is evident is that both risk and health communication have merged in acute ways. As Zhang and Centola (2019) suggest, the confluence of scientific and healthcare debates, economic and politic scenarios, technological and mediated environments, or social and cultural norms evidences how a pandemic becomes a privileged laboratory for observing the social contagion and cultural interdependencies at stake. Although the overlaps and gaps point to lessons to be learned in terms of routes and challenges, these shared responsibilities should also include recognition of the Latin cultural dispositions of Spain and Italy as a whole way of living, managing and informing risks.

References

Aguilar M and Bleda JM (2016) The healthcare system in Spain: from decentralization to economic current crisis. *Sociology and Anthropology* 4 (5): 306–314.

Arango C (2020) Lessons learned from the coronavirus health crisis in Madrid, Spain: how COVID-19 has changed our lives in the last 2 weeks. *Biological Psychiatry* 88 (7). Retrieved from https://www.biologicalpsychiatryjournal.com/article/S0006-3223(20)31493-1/fulltext (accessed 12 January 2021).

Avaaz (2020) How Facebook can flatten the curve of the coronavirus infodemic. Retrieved from https://secure.avaaz.org/campaign/en/facebook_coronavirus_misinformation (accessed 14 June 2020).

Barello S, Palamenghi L and Graffigna G (2020) Burnout and somatic symptoms among frontline healthcare professionals at the peak of the Italian COVID-19 pandemic.

Psychiatry Research 290. Retrieved from https://www.sciencedirect.com/science/article/abs/pii/S0165178120311975?via%3Dihub (accessed 12 January 2021).

Boholm A (2015) *Anthropology and Risk*. New York: Routledge.

Capano G (2020) Policy design and state capacity in the COVID-19 emergency in Italy: if you are not prepared for the (un)expected, you can be only what you already are. *Policy and Society* 39 (3): 326–344.

Carrascosa LL (2015) Ageing population and family support in Spain. *Journal of Comparative Family Studies* 46 (4): 499–516.

Carter DP and May PJ (2020) Making sense of the U.S. COVID-19 pandemic response: a policy regime perspective. *Administrative Theory & Praxis*, 42 (2): 265–277.

Chung A and Rimal RN (2016) Social norms: a review. *Review of Communication Research* 4: 1–28.

Dingwall R, Hoffman LM and Staniland K (2013) Introduction: why a *sociology* of pandemics? *Sociology of Health & Illness* 35 (2): 167–173.

European External Action Service (2020) COVID-19 disinformation. Retrieved from https://euvsdisinfo.eu (accessed 14 June 2020).

European Commission (2017) Attitudes towards the impact of digitisation and automation on daily life. Retrieved from http://ec.europa.eu/commfrontoffice/publicopinion/index.cfm/Survey/getSurveyDetail/instruments/SPECIAL/surveyKy/2160 (accessed 14 June 2020).

Eurostat (2020) Elderly population across EU regions. *Eurostat*, 2 April.

Ferraresi M (2020) Italy's politicians are making the coronavirus crisis worse. Retrieved from https://foreignpolicy.com/2020/03/09/italy-covid19-coronavirus-conte-salvini-epidemic-politicians-are-making-crisis-worse (accessed 1 September 2020).

García AA, García AA, Díaz JP and Rodríguez RP (2018) *Un perfil de las personas mayores en España, 2018: Indicadores estadísticos básicos*. Report no. 17, February. Madrid: Envejecimiento en red. Retrieved from http://envejecimiento.csic.es/documentos/documentos/enred-indicadoresbasicos2019.pdf

Geber S and Hefner D (2019) Social norms as communicative phenomena: a communication perspective on the theory of normative social behavior. *Studies in Communication and Media* 8: 6–28.

Giarelli G (2020) The governance of resilience. how the health systems have coped with the COVID-19 pandemic. *Culture e Studi del Sociale* 5 (1): 245–257.

Granovetter MS (1973) The strength of weak ties. *The American Journal of Sociology* 78 (6): 1360–1380.

Lapinski MK and Rimal RN (2005) An explication of social norms. *Communication Theory* 15 (2): 127–147.

Lee S, Hwang C and Moon MJ (2020) Policy learning and crisis policy-making: quadruple-loop learning and COVID-19 responses in South Korea. *Policy and Society* 39 (3): 363–381.

Legido-Quigley H, Mateos-García JT, Campos VR, Gea-Sánchez M, Muntaner C and McKee M (2020) The resilience of the Spanish health system against the COVID-19 pandemic. *The Lancet: Public Health* 5 (5). Retrieved from https://www.thelancet.com/journals/lanpub/article/PIIS2468-2667(20)300608/fulltext (accessed 12 January 2021).

Litwin H (2009) Social networks and well-being: a comparison of older people in mediterranean and non-Mediterranean countries. *The Journals of Gerontology: Series B* 65B (5): 599–608.

Lovari A (2020) Spreading (dis)trust: Covid-19 misinformation and government intervention in Italy. *Media and Communication* 8 (2): 458–461.

Lovari A, Martino V and Righetti N (2021) Blurred shots: investigating the information crisis around vaccination in Italy. *American Behavioral Scientist* 65 (2): 351–370.

Lupton D (2013) Risk and emotion: towards an alternative theoretical perspective. *Health, Risk & Society* 15 (8): 634–647.

Miller LJ and Lu W (2018) These are the economies with the most (and least) efficient health care. Retrieved from www.bloomberg.com/news/articles/2018-09-19/u-s-near-bottom-of-health-index-hong-kong-and-singapore-at-top (accessed 10 August 2020).

Moore SHE and Burgess A (2011) Risk rituals? *Journal of Risk Research* 14 (1): 111–124.

Naldini M (2003) *The Family in the Mediterranean Welfare States*. New York: Routledge.

Pan American Health Organization (2020) Understanding the infodemic and misinformation in the fight against COVID-19. Retrieved from https://iris.paho.org/bitstream/handle/10665.2/52052/Factsheet-infodemic_eng.pdf (accessed 10 August 2020).

Pavolini E and Vicarelli G (2013) Italy: A strange NHS with its paradoxes. In: Pavolini E and Guillén AM (eds) *Health Care Systems in Europe under Austerity*. Basingstoke: Palgrave, pp. 81–101.

Petmesidou M, Pavolini E and Guillén AM (2014) South European healthcare systems under harsh austerity: a progress–regression mix? *South European Society and Politics* 19 (3): 331–352.

Rahman A and Jahan Y (2020) Defining a 'risk group' and ageism in the era of COVID-19. *Journal of Loss and Trauma* 25 (8): 631–634.

Rhodes T and Lancaster K (2020) Mathematical models as public troubles in COVID-19 infection control: following the numbers. *Health Sociology Review* 29 (2): 177–194.

Rimal RN and Lapinski MK (2009) Why health communication is important in public health. *Bulletin of the World Health Organization* 87 (4): 247.

Rutter H, Wolpert M and Greenhalgh T (2020) Managing uncertainty in the covid-19 era. Available at: https://blogs.bmj.com/bmj/2020/07/22/managing-uncertainty-in-the-covid-19-era/ (accessed 1 September 2020).

Salaverría R, Buslón N, López-Pan F, León B, López-Goñi I and Erviti MC (2020) Desinformación en tiempos de pandemia: tipología de los bulos sobre la COVID-19. *El Profesional de la Información* 29 (3): e290315.

Sánchez-García JJ (2019) Catorce años de implantación de la salud digital en España: dónde estamos y dónde deberíamos estar. Available at: https://empresas.blogthinkbig.com/implantacion-de-la-salud-digital-en-espana-balance-de-catorce-anos/ (accessed 14 June 2020).

Scambler G (2020) Covid-19 as a 'breaching experiment': exposing the fractured society. *Health Sociology Review* 29 (2): 140–148.

Serapioni M (2018) Sistemi sanitari e disuguaglianze di salute. L'impatto della crisi nei Paesi mediterranei. *Sociologia Italiana* 12: 187–201.

Serapioni M and Hespanha P (2019) Crisis and austerity in southern europe: impact on economies and societies. *e-cadernos CES* 31: 4–18.

Soper GA (1919) The lessons of the pandemic. *Science* 49: 501–506.

United Nations (2019) *Living Arrangements of Older Persons around the World*. Report for the Department of Economic and Social Affairs. Report no. 2019/2, April. New York: United Nations.

Vaccari C (2012) Online participation in Italy. In: Anduiza E, Jensen MJ and Jorba L (eds) *Digital Media and Political Engagement Worldwide*. New York: Cambridge University Press, pp. 138–159.

Walter N, Murphy ST, Frank LB and Ball-Rokeach SJ (2019) The power of brokerage: case study of normative behavior, Latinas and cervical cancer. *Communication Research* 46 (5): 639–662.

Wong CML and Jensen O (2020) The paradox of trust: perceived risk and public compliance during the COVID-19 pandemic in Singapore. *Journal of Risk Research* 23 (7–8): 1021–1030.

Wright KB (2016) Communication in health-related online social support groups/communities: a review of research on predictors of participation, applications of social support theory, and health outcomes. *Review of Communication Research* 4: 65–87.

Yabanci B (2020) Fuzzy borders between populism and sacralized politics: mission, leader, community and performance in 'new' Turkey. *Politics, Religion & Ideology* 21 (1): 92–112.

Zhang J and Centola D (2019) Social networks and health: new developments in diffusion, online and offline. *Annual Review of Sociology* 45: 9–109.

Zinn, J (2008) Heading into the unknown: everyday strategies for managing risk and uncertainty. *Health, Risk & Society* 10 (5): 439–450.

14

RISKY WORK

Providing healthcare in the age of COVID-19

Karen Willis and Natasha Smallwood

Introduction

The story of the international coronavirus pandemic is by now well known. The lives of people across the globe were transformed almost overnight from the beginning of 2020, as the virus spread. Coexisting with the threat of infection was governments' need to ensure that health facilities were able to cope with the onslaught of cases, including those requiring intensive care and possibly ventilation. In early 2020, frightening images from across the globe of overcrowded hospitals and the establishment of field hospitals provided graphic indicators of the consequences of rapid coronavirus spread. Such images coexisted with emerging stories of strain on healthcare workers and statistics indicating high rates of infection and death in the health workforce.

This information provided the backdrop against which health services in Australia engaged in a medical surge event to ensure adequate pandemic preparation. Frontline healthcare workers at high risk of exposure to pandemic illnesses in hospitals and the community have had to respond quickly to many challenges, including: escalating workloads; large volumes of new information; new work practices and roles; upskilling in the diagnosis and care of patients with COVID-19; being redeployed or facing job insecurity: and changes in their social setting (social distancing, school closures and working from home). The impact of the anticipated threat was powerfully captured by an Australian current affairs television programme called 'Flattening the Curve' (Australian Broadcasting Corporation, 2020), including statements by health professionals such as: 'It's overwhelming especially being on the frontline' and 'It's like waiting for a ticking time bomb to come in'.

As the pandemic unfolded and Australia experienced much better control of COVID than many countries, it might have been expected that the stress experienced during the medical surge event would reduce as health professionals 'got on with the job' of managing the virus and the ensuing case load, which was much lower than many international settings. But this was not the case. Just three weeks after easing of the lockdown restrictions introduced across the country in late March 2020, one Australian state (Victoria) experienced a second wave of cases, necessitating the re-introduction of strict lockdown restrictions across the state, particularly in Australia's second largest city, Melbourne. With health services back on high alert (but still managing the case load) the combination of increased stress and anxiety, changed work conditions and changes in social arrangements appear to have overwhelmed many frontline health professionals. Personal risk of catching the coronavirus was only one of their fears.

In this chapter, we tease out the interwoven risks and psychosocial impacts of health work during the pandemic. We draw on preliminary findings from free-text responses in a survey of over 9,000 healthcare workers in Australia, which illustrate issues related to workplace disruption, healthcare delivery challenges that result in moral injury, and concerns of being simultaneously at risk and risky which necessitate the development of new strategies to manage work, home and family.

Working and the age of COVID

The impact on working arrangements and conditions has been one of the most dramatic social effects of the pandemic (Cohen, 2020; Stephens et al., 2020). In Australia, working from home (for those who could) became the 'new normal' (Sander, 2020). The closing of schools was accompanied by the requirement for parents to homeschool their children, with the gendered impact of this for working parents particularly noted (Ruppanner et al., 2020). These changes were unevenly spread – with rapid change and increased pace in some sectors and high unemployment in others.

The healthcare sector was one of the sectors that was placed under high pressure. The pandemic has emerged at a time when there was already clear evidence that health professionals experience high risks of poor mental health in their everyday work environment. Mental health difficulties, stress and burnout in health practitioners are widely reported, with rates increasing over time (Karimi et al., 2016; Dzau et al., 2018; Omar et al., 2015). Doctors and nurses have higher rates of burnout, depression, anxiety and suicide than other occupations (Petrie et al., 2019). While less is known about other groups of clinicians, early studies are troubling (Courtney et al., 2013). These issues have consequences, not just for the practitioners themselves but for the wider health service, as poor mental health of clinicians affects quality of clinical care (Tawfik et al., 2019) patient safety, and workforce retention and engagement (Salyers et al., 2015).

For those working in an already high-stress environment, crisis events such as pandemics represent a tipping point for those frontline workers already vulnerable to mental health problems. Evidence from previous pandemics such as the severe acute respiratory syndrome (SARS) in 2003 indicates a 'substantial negative effect on a statistically significant' number of healthcare workers (Maunder et al., 2006).

A survey of Chinese health professionals about the impact of the COVID crisis (Lai et al., 2020) found an increased psychological burden, with frontline healthcare workers being particularly vulnerable, especially nursing staff and healthcare workers with family responsibilities. Along with heightened psychological distress, the perception of risk, rather than direct exposure, is implicated in increased psychological illness (Tam et al., 2004). Particular issues identified as resulting from the psychosocial impact of crisis events such as pandemics are: anxiety about personal exposure to increased risk in the workplace (Gallagher and Schleyer, 2020); transmission of risk to families and loved ones (Nickell et al., 2004); community stigmatisation of healthcare workers as virus carriers (Jayawardena, 2020; Nguyen, 2020); working outside their normal scope of practice (Nickell et al., 2004); and organisational factors, including limited resources forcing rationing of care (Lai et al., 2020).

Despite the well-documented occupational risks of healthcare work, the risks are rarely acknowledged in the public sphere. The focus tends more often to be on the risks experienced by patients or clients, rather than those who deliver healthcare services (Gale et al., 2016). Adding to the complexity of focusing on healthcare workers is the need to examine the permeable boundaries between work and home, as risks may not always be contained in one sphere. Thus, gaining insight into the home and work interplay is a vital but often overlooked aspect of occupational health and wellbeing (Baxter and Alexander, 2008).

The concept of 'spillover' is one way of understanding the way in which these two domains intersect. Usually applied to the way that stress is transmitted between home and work roles, spillover refers to 'the means by which behaviours, attitudes, and experiences in one environment spill over or affect other environments that an individual occupies on a daily basis' (Dilworth, 2004: 241). The case of the COVID pandemic highlights spillover for healthcare workers in a different way: they are simultaneously a source of danger and risk to others in one domain (within the family sphere), and in the other domain are 'at risk' and needing protection (at work). In this context, these workers are faced with negotiating dual demands, often where there is uncertainty about the danger they are navigating. As Polgar argues, 'risk and risk perception are transformed through interpretive processes inside and outside of different occupational contexts' (2000: 254). Thus, in a pandemic, risk perception for healthcare workers is shaped not only by the organisational approach to safety, but also by social factors relating to transmission.

A further dimension of healthcare workers' experience relates to how changed work practices impact on how they undertake their caring roles, job satisfaction and the value they feel they are contributing. There is now also greater attention to the concept of 'moral injury' (McKinnon and Lanius, 2020) as it relates to healthcare workers. Previously applied most commonly to the contradictions faced by defence forces, moral injury occurs when one's deeply held beliefs or values are in conflict with the actions one is required to take. Examples in healthcare include the rationing of care when resources are in short supply or being unable to provide the quality of care due to the constraints of wearing personal protective equipment

(PPE). Being unable to allow family members at the bedside of dying patients may also be experienced as moral injury.

Our study: future-proofing the frontline

Our online anonymous survey of frontline healthcare workers in Australia aimed to identify the psychological, social and occupational impacts of COVID. We invited workers from a range of occupations (doctors, nurses, allied health, paramedics and clerical workers) across a range of settings (hospitals, primary care, private care) to complete an online anonymous survey focused on their personal responses, as well as their perceptions about workplace responses to the pandemic. At the time of writing, over 9,000 healthcare workers had taken the survey. Respondents were predominantly from the state of Victoria (87%) (reflecting our own location in that state and the networks we used to recruit participants), were more likely to be female (81%) and just over half (55%) were aged between 20 and 40 years. Most respondents (82%) worked in public metropolitan hospitals.

The survey revealed high levels of self-reported anxiety, stress and burnout, and low use of mental health services. Over half the respondents (56%) were worried about infecting their family with COVID. While scales, instruments and closed-ended responses are excellent in measuring prevalence and attitudes to various phenomena, an explicit strategy to generate free-text responses can elicit rich information about respondents' experiences (O'Cathain and Thomas, 2004). For this reason, we used targeted open-ended questions to gain deeper insights into respondents' experiences. The final survey question asked: 'Is there anything else that you would like to tell us about the impact of the COVID-19 pandemic or regarding supports that you feel are useful for wellbeing?'. Approximately one-quarter of the respondents provided free-text data in response to this question. Many of their responses focus on the changes at work and in their personal lives. Taking the first 300 substantive responses (for example, we removed those who simply responded, 'no' or 'thank you for doing this survey'), we undertook an exploratory overview of the key concerns identified by healthcare workers in response to this question. We were particularly concerned to understand how they expressed the notion of disruption to social and work life, along with perceptions of risk and strategies to mitigate risk.

Findings

The responses to the free-text question were broad ranging and covered three diverse areas. First, participants used the opportunity to share information about the wellbeing strategies that have proved helpful during the pandemic, including activities such as yoga and mindfulness, connecting with family and friends and the supports that they gain from their peers. Second, they also highlighted the importance of organisation or public policy specific roles responding to the pandemic. The third set of responses is the focus of this chapter: the information they provided about how the pandemic has affected them personally; the idea of being both 'a risk' and 'at risk'; and their thoughts about being a healthcare worker during pandemic times.

Disruption and guilt

As was the case for other essential workers and those who remained in the workforce generally, healthcare workers experienced disruptions to their everyday life. They often discussed an effect of spillover between family and work, as encapsulated by this comment:

> People working in front line healthcare who are trying to do their best in a rapidly changing landscape, are also impacted by effects on family, home schooling, elderly relatives and basic day to day issues (e.g. can't buy basics because of 8 p.m. curfew in Victoria). The pandemic affects every aspect of our lives and is impossible to get away from.

There were also references to the gendered impact of profound change experienced along with the personal sense of risk, with descriptions of how spillover from work affected family and opportunities for self-care.

> One major negative has been on my days off I should be looking after my 4 and 10 year old daughters but I am so distracted by emails, phone calls from distressed staff, extra work, trying to source masks, Zoom meeting etc. etc., that my children have suffered. I have also had to increase my on-call workload that means staying all weekend at a hotel close to the hospital. I have had way less time to exercise and do stuff that relaxes me, or just have time out. There are so many issues, I just focus on what needs to be done next. Ultimately my children are suffering now. However the most important thing is that they have a mother that is healthy at the end of all of this.

For many respondents, the pandemic brought a heightened level of fear and sense of vulnerability which was new to them:

> I feel physically vulnerable and threatened when outside the house. I've previously only felt this way when physically threatened or in a dangerous situation.
>
> I feel for the first time ever, that I have mental health fragility. Even recognising that, I find stressful.
>
> I have never in my life had the feeling of impending doom and severe anxiety before March this year.

> COVID-19 has impacted my well being for the first time in my career in Palliative Care. I hadn't realised how much until I took a step back (on leave) and talked with other health professionals about how I was feeling.

Additionally, the feeling of guilt was expressed frequently. It was apparent that respondents felt a disruption to their usual disposition of caring and curing in their professional role. The pandemic forced them to think and feel differently about what they could contribute professionally:

> I feel guilty because at my age I do not feel comfortable stepping forward into direct contact with COVID patients ... and then I get angry for feeling this way. I worked through both HIV and Hep C being lethal infections.
>
> I feel guilty all the time for not volunteering to do more but I don't feel safe at work because it is obvious healthcare worker protection is not adequately addressed, so I will not volunteer for work where my safety is not adequately addressed.

This feeling of guilt was also apparent when respondents tried to balance their anxiety alongside the fact that they still had a job, for which they should be 'grateful' when compared to the fate of others in the community:

> I feel sad that my job has changed so much and guilty about feeling this way as others have lost their jobs and/or loved ones.
>
> I am concerned about the impact of COVID-19 restrictions on patients' mental and physical health over the past 9 months and counting. I feel survivors' guilt – seeing patients who've lost livelihoods, have no reason to leave the house and are on the brink of complete breakdowns, *I feel terrible knowing I have a job, income, and on top of that I am hailed a hero, for no good reason* [emphasis added].

Respondents also experienced guilt when they were redeployed so that they weren't providing direct care to patients who may have tested positive to COVID. Furthermore, their responses indicate a struggle to weigh up the options of continuing to provide care to patients versus the risk that this choice may pose to themselves and their families:

> I felt guilty about ceasing work as a clinical emergency nurse initially but felt that I had a greater responsibility to my family to keep myself and them safe.
>
> I tried to work on a COVID ward but my anxiety for the wellbeing of my family (and providing for them financially, especially when thinking about quarantine which would not be remunerated), meant I couldn't do more than one shift. I was too stressed. ... I would like to contribute to the pandemic workforce, but my family comes first – both in terms of my physical presence, and me providing for them financially. I am sorry for this.

Vulnerability and risk choices

Evident across all responses was the struggle that respondents faced suddenly, feeling that they were both at risk and a risk to others. While healthcare workers face risk every day in their occupations, the uncertainty around the pandemic highlighted a risk that was felt to be less controllable than other more familiar risks. Furthermore, the publicising of cases ensured that there was constant and heightened community awareness about the virus. As one respondent stated: 'Going to work makes me feel unsafe everyday and the feeling varies according to the community transmission levels'. It is also evident that people worked hard to strategise according to their intersecting perceptions about risk. The first risk they articulated was that they were 'a risk' to others, particularly in relation to their interactions with family and friends. Many respondents indicated the strategies they had put in place due to this heightened sense of being 'a risk':

> [I'm] more worried about being a carer for my elderly mother than anything else. I do not want to accidently pass on the virus to my family especially mum.
>
> My siblings can help support my parents when I can't due to my increased risk.
>
> I am also worried about passing on the disease to my young children at home.
>
> I have 3 frontline healthcare workers in my family/household. This worries me. It increases the potential for this to get into my home and once one of us gets it, it will be hard to prevent the rest from getting it.

Respondents also reflected on community attitudes and their social networks, in which they were viewed as being risky:

> Our kids' tutors (e.g. piano and Chinese) cancelled their lessons before their peers. I couldn't help but think it was because we were HCWs [healthcare workers].
>
> I have seen friends on one occasion since March (who were also doctors) and we met up outdoors when the restrictions were eased. I have essentially become isolated because everyone else has been too concerned to meet up with me due to my job even during safer periods (e.g. telehealth-only work without direct patient contact).
>
> I was furloughed for 2 weeks, and had to move into an apartment temporarily, so as to not affect my family who were very worried that I could be detrimental to their health (they tried to hide it, but I could just tell).

The second way in which respondents discussed risk was being 'at risk'; again, personal strategies were mentioned, along with the need for protection in the workplace:

> I wrote a will this year. I really should have had one already, but a lot of nurses are now dead, so I wrote one.
>
> Huge anxiety, sleepless nights, writing a will to identify who was going to look after my 11-month-old baby if my husband and I both died.

These responses provide examples of the respondents' 'risk reasoning' and considered strategies that they would enact if they did test positive. Again there was a weighing up of the risks and the options available to them. The two contrasting perspectives are illustrated by these respondents:

> I'm very worried about the implications for my family if I contract COVID. We live in a very small unit without outdoor space. I have an 18-month-old [baby]. It will be almost impossible to isolate from him and my husband in our home. Despite the fact that I am aware I would be eligible for a hotel room, I do not think mentally that I could be separated from my child for that period of time. As such, we have decided that if I get COVID we will isolate in our small home together and it is likely my family will all contract the virus.
>
> I am completely unwilling to risk bringing COVID home to my family so I will have to personally pay for a hotel if I'm in that situation.

Being a healthcare worker in pandemic times

A third level of disruption was expressed by respondents as they considered what it meant to be a healthcare worker during rapid change. Here the free text related to the provision of appropriate resources to do their job in a safe manner and changes to the way that they were able to provide care to patients. Some reflected on whether they should remain in the health workforce. Others discussed how the pandemic was illuminating existing and ongoing issues with healthcare provision, rather than posing a new challenge.

Personal protective equipment as a signifier of value

One of the issues that emerged throughout all the responses is how provision of PPE contributes to both personal feelings of safety and trust in the healthcare institution. As Smith (2020) states: 'perceived adequacy of PPE and infection control procedures in healthcare workplaces is associated with important differences in anxiety and depression symptoms'. Reflections on workplace provision of PPE were frequent, with respondents articulating how inadequate provision made them feel as a worker, as illustrated in the following:

> I am reluctant to work at my job without adequate protection or without it being a priority to protect HCWs [healthcare workers]. The reactive response

> to biohazard risk, the numbers of staff infected in Australia. *I feel expendable* [emphasis added].

> I am angered by being constantly offered wellbeing programmes by employer and government authorities instead of Tier 3 PPE/fit testing and training. The elephant in the room is that many of us are worried about life and death survival of us and our families from COVID-19 infection, and they want me to meditate and do crafts!

> I have felt powerless over my own safety and that of my family. I feel I have been forced to work in an unsafe manner due to lack of PPE and as a result *feel dispensable* and my safety and welfare have been completely disregarded by management and the public health system. I have compared this feeling to what it must have felt like for young men being conscripted to war [emphasis added].

Patients and patient care

Changes in work practices affected the delivery of care, and respondents commented on how well they felt they could do their job of providing care in a new environment, as well as the impacts for patients from reduced contact with family due to visitor restrictions, and reduced contact with healthcare workers due to working in PPE. Respondents felt compromised, or experienced a form of 'moral injury', in their capacity to provide care. For some, it was about job satisfaction, as illustrated by this comment: 'Minimised patient contacted has resulted in reduced job satisfaction'. Other participants voiced their concern at the visitor restrictions that healthcare settings imposed:

> Overwhelming sadness. The manner of death for these patients all alone.

> Not letting family and relatives be with their sick relatives is the hardest thing about COVID. I think we could be more flexible in our approach.

> I hate that patients aren't allowed to have visitors. Especially a lot of the general medicine patients have cognitive impairment, or they are close to end of life without being in the last week of life, or their English isn't the first language, and their care and hospital experience would be so much better if they were allowed a visitor to help them understand the treatment plan during ward rounds and encourage them to eat at meal times.

The third idea relating to patient issues focused on the capacity to provide high quality care for all patients, not just those with COVID:

> I worry that on balance of things, overall more harm will come to patients by having inferior medical care provided than from the risk of COVID.

> My biggest anxieties have been around stock shortages (especially with critical theatre and oncology products – because if they're not available and there are no alternatives, the patient can't receive treatment, what are the ramifications of that? Will the patient be worse off, will I be in trouble with the patient, their family, the medical staff, the hospital, the pharmacy?)

Choosing to do health work in pandemic times

While there are some respondents who saw the pandemic as a time when they could contribute positively during a crisis, overwhelmingly respondents indicated a high level of stress felt during this time. The views below are indicative of the feelings that healthcare workers expressed:

> I have never worked this hard, or experienced this degree of stress or emotional toll from the work I have been doing the last 2 months. During the height of the pandemic, I had hoped I would get COVID so I would not have to come to work.
>
> Less often do I look forward to work. Almost every day I think about how much I don't want to be a nurse and how life would be easier in so many other jobs.

Linked to the ideas about disruption to self and risk discussed above are comments throughout the responses indicating that healthcare workers are reconsidering their career options. Appearing frequently throughout the free-text responses are references to the fact that healthcare workers don't feel adequately compensated for the risks that they face; the thoughts of career change are inextricably linked to respondents' perceptions about being valued in the workplace:

> I am considering taking time away from work, as I don't feel well compensated for the risks and effort.
>
> Being a junior doctor is hard enough. The pandemic has made me want to quit medicine even after spending most of my life striving towards being a doctor. I'm having a really hard time.
>
> The pandemic has affected my outlook so much that I even imagine pursing an alternate career … It just feels like we are sacrificing ourselves without any compensation and to be told we signed up for this is unhelpful. Our lives matter too.

Disrupted workplace or more of the same?

Finally, throughout the free text is commentary about the state of healthcare provision; with many respondents reporting on the stresses of being a healthcare worker, which already existed but have now come under the spotlight during the pandemic. These final comments are illustrative of the perception of a system under stress, as well as healthcare workers' experiences of stress. Many respondents emphasised the importance of a system-wide approach to providing a safe workplace, rather than a focus on individuals who experience stress resulting from a crisis:

> COVID hasn't caused any new problems it has merely highlighted all the pre-existing inadequacies of the healthcare system and society in general.
>
> COVID 19 has highlighted how burnt out and stressed junior doctors are at baseline, a pandemic had added considerable stress to an already stressful roster for many.
>
> It would be great if the support that nurses received and the acknowledgement of all the things we do was all the time and not only because there is a pandemic.
>
> We're all just exhausted. I was burnt out pre-pandemic and now feel so guilty about wanting to leave medicine and will stay because I feel I need to, not because it's what's best for me.

Conclusion

The early information about COVID was that it provided an apparently indiscriminate and invisible risk across the whole community. While at a community level this may have been the case, the consequences for actively contributing to the fight against this virus magnified the risk felt and experienced by many healthcare workers. As healthcare workers are also social beings, they experienced a 'perfect storm' of both social and workplace disruption, resulting in descriptions of the negative effects of spillover. The scale of disruption that they experienced occurred at multiple levels; in effect, it was impossible to escape the pandemic. The issue of PPE provision was more than just about the materials that healthcare workers needed to do their job safely; it was a major signifier of perceived personal value to the organisation. Similarly, the contingent nature of risk that emerged, as respondents considered both their own vulnerability, the risk they posed to others and their consequent decision, was also, for many, about the responsibilities of the workplace.

For many workers across the globe, delineations between home and work have increasingly blurred in physical terms, as working from home became the norm. In the case of healthcare workers, this blurring of boundaries (or spillover) became a pivotal point around which the negotiation about risk occurred, as they considered how their being 'at risk' in their workplace made them 'a risk' to their family. Already at risk of occupationally induced issues of anxiety and burnout, the pandemic brought about changes in practice and in risk that exacerbated feelings of stress and anxiety. What emerges most from the disruptive effects we have described above is the significance of feeling valued (or not) in the workplace. While respondents also described a range of individual-level strategies that they engaged during the pandemic to support their health and wellbeing, and to mitigate their risk, many of them articulated the need for workplace and structural remedies, rather than exhortations for individuals to take care of themselves (which was often the messaging they reported from their workplaces). As this sentiment was evident across the range of ideas that were expressed, it is fitting that we conclude with the words of the following respondent:

> I really think the most important thing is how Australia manages the COVID-19 pandemic and what our employers' attitude to occupational health and safety is. Everything else – all the individual level interventions like yoga apps – are chicken feed in comparison. There is a big risk that focusing on the individual-level strategies lets governments and employers 'off the hook' and frames any distress as the worker's fault.

Acknowledgements

We wish to thank the Royal Melbourne Hospital Foundation for providing funding for the survey and the frontline health workers who generously took time to complete the survey.

References

Australian Broadcasting Corporation (2020) Flattening the curve. *Four Corners* [television programme], 4 May. Retrieved from www.abc.net.au/4corners/flattening-the-curve/12213506 (accessed 12 October 2020).

Baxter J and Alexander M (2008) Mother's work-to-family strain in single and couple parent families: the role of job characteristics and support. *Australian Journal of Social Issues* 43 (2): 195–214.

Cohen L (2020) The coronavirus is changing how we work – possibly permanently. *The Conversation*, 26 March. Retrieved from https://theconversation.com/the-coronavirus-is-changing-how-we-work-possibly-permanently-134344 (accessed 12 October 2020).

Courtney J, Francis A and Paxton S (2013) Caring for the country: fatigue, sleep and mental health in Australian rural paramedic shift workers. *Journal of Community Health* 38 (1): 178–186.

Dilworth JEL (2004) Predictors of negative spillover from family to work. *Journal of Family Studies* 25 (2): 241–261.

Dzau VJ, Kirch DG and Nasca TJ (2018) To care is human: collectively confronting the clinician-burnout crisis. *New England Journal of Medicine* 378 (4): 312–314.

Gale NK, Thomas GM, Thwaites R, Greenfield S and Brown P (2016) Towards a sociology of risk work: a narrative review and synthesis, *Sociology Compass* 10 (11): 1046–1071.

Gallagher TH and Schleyer AM (2020) 'We signed up for this!' Student and trainee responses to the Covid-19 pandemic. *New England Journal of Medicine* 382. Retrieved from https://www.nejm.org/doi/full/10.1056/NEJMp2005234 (accessed 13 January 2021).

Jayawardena A (2020) Waiting for something positive. *New England Journal of Medicine* 382. Retrieved from https://www.nejm.org/doi/full/10.1056/NEJMp2008797 (accessed 13 January 2021).

Karimi L, Leggatt S, Cheng C, Donohue L, Bartram T and Oakman J (2016) Are organisational factors impacting the emotional withdrawal of community nurses? *Australian Health Review* 41 (4): 359–364.

Lai J, Ma S and Wang Y (2020) Factors associated with mental health outcomes among health care workers exposed to coronavirus disease 2019. *JAMA Network Open* 3 (3). Retrieved from https://jamanetwork.com/journals/jamanetworkopen/fullarticle/2763229 (13 January 2021).

Maunder R, Lancee WJ and Wasylenki A (2006) Long-term psychological and occupational effects of providing hospital health-care during SARS outbreak. *Emerging Infectious Diseases* 12 (12): 1924–1932.

McKinnon M and Lanius R (2020) Hard choices put health workers at risk of mental anguish, PTSD during coronavirus. *The Conversation*, 15 May. Retrieved from https://theconversation.com/hard-choices-put-health-workers-at-risk-of-mental-anguish-ptsd-during-coronavirus-136812 (accessed 12 October 2020).

Nickell LA, Crighton EJ, Tracy CS, Al-Enazy H, Bolaji Y, Hanjrah S, Hussain A, Makhlouf S and Upshur RE (2004) Psychosocial effects of SARS on hospital staff: survey of a large tertiary care institution. *Canadian Medical Association Journal* 170 (5): 7893–7898.

Nguyen K (2020) NSW nurses told not wear scrubs outside of hospital due to abuse over coronavirus fears. *ABC News*, 5 April. Retrieved from www.abc.net.au/news/2020-04-05/nsw-nurses-midwives-abused-during-coronavirus-pandemic/12123216 (accessed 8 October 2020).

O'Cathain A and Thomas KJ (2004) 'Any other comments?' Open questions on questionnaires – a bane or a bonus to research? *BMC Medical Research Methodology* 4 (1): 1–7.

Omar A, Elmaraghi S, Mahmoud M, Khalil M, Singh R and Ostowski P (2015), Impact of leadership on ICU clinicians' burnout. *Critical Care Medicine* 18 (3): 139.

Petrie K, Crawford J, Baker S, Dean K, Robinson J and Veness B (2019) Interventions to reduce symptoms of common mental disorders and suicidal ideation in physicians: a systematic review and meta-analysis. *The Lancet Psychiatry* 6 (3): 225–234.

Polgar M (2000) Concern, caution, and care: HIV risk perception among hospital nurses. *Sociological Inquiry* 70 (3): 253–279.

Ruppanner L, Collins C and Scarborough W (2020) COVID-19 is a disaster for mothers' employment. And no, working from home is not the solution. *The Conversation*, 21 July. Retrieved from https://theconversation.com/covid-19-is-a-disaster-for-mothers-employment-and-no-working-from-home-is-not-the-solution-142650 (accessed 12 October 2020).

Sander L (2020) Coronavirus could spark a revolution in working from home. Are we ready? *The Conversation*, 11 March. Retrieved from https://theconversation.com/coronavirus-could-spark-a-revolution-in-working-from-home-are-we-ready-133070 (accessed 12 October 2020).

Smith P (2020) Health-care workers lacking PPE suffer more from anxiety and depression. *The Conversation*, 29 September. Retrieved from https://theconversation.com/heath-care-workers-lacking-ppe-suffer-from-more-anxiety-and-depression-145612 (accessed 12 October 2020).

Stephens K, Jahn LS, Fox S, Charoensap-Kelly P, Mitra R, Sutton J, Waters E, Xie B and Meisenbach R (2020) Collective sensemaking around COVID-19: experiences, concerns and agendas for our rapidly changing organisational lives. *Management Communication Quarterly* 343 (3): 426–457.

Tam C, Pang E, Lam L and Chiu H (2004) Severe acute respiratory syndrome (SARS) in Hong Kong in 2003: stress and psychological impact among frontline workers. *Psychological Medicine* 34 (7): 1197–1204.

Tawfik DS, Scheid A, Profit J, Shanafeit T, Trackel M, Adair K, Sexton JB and Ioannidis J (2019) Evidence relating health-care provider burnout and quality of care: a systematic review and meta-analysis. *Annals of Internal Medicine* 171 (8): 555–567.

Salyers M, Flanagan M, Firmin R and Rolling A (2015) Clinicians' perceptions of how burnout affects their work. *Psychiatric Services* 66 (2): 204–207.

PART V

Marginalisation and discrimination

15

THE PLIGHT OF THE PARENT-CITIZEN?

Examples of resisting (self-)responsibilisation and stigmatisation by Dutch Muslim parents and organisations during the COVID-19 crisis

Alex Schenkels, Sakina Loukili and Paul Mutsaers

Introduction

When the Dutch government announced the temporary closure of public spaces like schools, kindergartens and mosques on 15 March 2020 in response to the COVID-19 outbreak, Dutch Muslim families found themselves being responsibilised in areas such as home schooling, homeworking and home praying and feasting. At the same time, the outbreak has exacerbated racial discrimination, inequalities and (public) stigma (Pang, 2020). Dutch media reports have framed Muslims as a risk group, once again, in pandemic times (Slaats, 2020). Combined, these developments have further intensified the parenting challenges for Muslim families.

Elsewhere, we have described how Dutch Muslim parents have internalised, negotiated *and* reconstructed intensive parenting norms (Schenkels and Mutsaers, 2019). These norms concern questions of child centrality, family responsibility, expert guidance, emotional labour and other matters long since known to be the essentials of intensive parenting (Hays, 1996). In this chapter, which is based on the doctoral studies of two of the authors, we discuss what has (not) changed with the coming of the COVID pandemic, by focusing on both pandemic-related (and intensifying) struggles within Muslim families (study 1) and on the role of Muslim organisations in cushioning the (racist) blow for these families (study 2).

In what follows, we first sketch a brief and inevitably selective history of Muslim families and organisations in the Netherlands, focusing in particular on the notion of intensive parenting in relation to our studies. We then present the COVID-related data from the first study, by examining how Dutch Muslim parents find each other online for (spiritual) support, particularly in relation to home schooling. Our findings suggest that while intensive parenting is developing into 'hyper-intensive' parenting, it is being challenged by these parents. However, in our discussion of the second study, we present more serious signs of resistance, specifically against the intensive parenting ideal of family resilience in the face of social ills such as racism (cf. Faircloth and Murray, 2015). Whereas the intensive parenting ideology spurs images of the 'parent-citizen' who takes responsibility and is seen as the source of and solution to all kinds of social problems (Edwards, Gillies and Horsely, 2013), to be dealt with in the private sphere, we see new developments in the public sphere, where Muslim organisations present themselves as an extended family helping to mitigate the effects of racism against Muslim families. In presenting findings from both projects, we argue for the importance of 'public pedagogy', particularly in pandemic times.

Muslim families and organisations in the (COVID-affected) Netherlands

Muslims form the largest yet most stigmatised minority group in the Netherlands, making up roughly five per cent of the population (Maliepaard and Alba, 2016). Within this group, most second- and third-generation migrants have a background in Turkey or Morocco, from which their parents migrated to the Netherlands as 'guest workers' from the 1960s onwards. Unlike their parents, second- and third-generation Muslims can benefit from a broad range of Islamic organisations in politics, education, health and youth care that are now more firmly embedded in Dutch society than before. The present situation is very different from the early days of Dutch multiculturalism, in which migrant organisations existed in 'splendid isolation' because of the typical structure of Dutch 'pillar society'(Slootman, 2017), where this society was shaped by a strong commitment to a common ideology and shared values. New organisations like NIDA and IPeP (Islamic Pedagogy and Psychology Practices), studied by us in our two doctoral projects, are mostly run by young, higher-educated Muslims. These organisations are known to play a key role in the emergence and emancipation of a Muslim middle class in Dutch society (Slootman, 2017). NIDA, an Islamic political party currently led by the pedagogue Nourdin el Ouali, was founded in 2013 to give a voice to new generations of Muslims (in the Qur'anic context, *nida* means 'call'). IPeP was also founded in 2013 to provide an Islamic alternative in care and parenting support for Dutch Muslims (Islamic Pedagogy and Psychology Practices, 2020). As the findings below demonstrate, these trends towards emancipation and integration also mean that new generations of Muslim parents have begun to adopt (and adapt) intensive parenting practices and discourses that were once primarily practised by white middle-class families (Rollock et al., 2014).

Intensive parenting is described as parenting that is 'child-centred, expert guided, emotionally absorbing, labour-intensive, and financially expensive' (Hays, 1996: 8). It is typically oriented towards the nuclear family and encourages parents to think of the family as a project to be managed and of the child as a 'profitable investment' that, if endowed with the right education and concerted cultivation by its parents, is moulded into an entrepreneurial self (Güney-Frahm, 2020). Intensive parenting is (part of) a dominant ideology because it is built up of systems of representation setting the 'limits to the degree to which a society-in-dominance can easily, smoothly, and functionally reproduce itself' (Hall, 1985: 113). Keeping within these limits is important for ideologies to persist, since it renders them invisible, self-evident, and normalised – key features for the survival of ideologies (Blommaert, 2005).

Previous generations of Muslim parents parented using (inward-looking) extended family structures for support and guidance (Rezai, 2017). This parenting model differed from the atomistic parent–child relation that is a widespread norm in western Europe and believed to be key to the optimum development of the child (Faircloth and Murray, 2015). Although it has been argued that preoccupation with their children's academic success has affected parents in western Europe less than their Asian or American counterparts (Ochs and Kremer-Sadlik, 2015), the idea of parents being the central responsible agent for their children to thrive and succeed is internalised in Dutch culture as well (Geigner, Vandenbroek and Roets, 2014). However, like their non-Muslim Dutch counterparts, contemporary Muslim parents tend to be more concerned with the parent–child dyad, school performance management and child centricity (Pels and de Gruijter, 2006) and take their concerns online, where parenting is publicly portrayed and performed (Schenkels and Mutsaers, 2019). Despite evidence of negative effects on (minority) families (Rollock et al., 2014), intensive parenting has been largely unquestioned. Befitting a successful ideology, its internal contradictions have been diminished; for example, between parental determinism and expert guidance, best captured by the sentence 'trust your instincts, but let us tell you what those instincts should be' (Faircloth and Murray, 2015: 1120).

Parenting hyper-intensified: the self-responsibilisation reflex

Once the COVID crisis had begun to exert effects in Europe and children were sent home to continue education there, we encountered a steady flow of COVID-related posts as part of an ongoing (n)ethnographic study of Dutch Islamic parenting Facebook and Instagram pages. The online sharing of parental experiences peaked in the first days after the schools closed. We analysed a selection of social media pages (those of IPeP, Kleine Moslims and Fatimama), selected because they seemed the most active between mid-March and August 2020 and most focused on the subject under consideration, compared to other relevant sites and blogs. Additionally, we held seven interviews and conducted six open-ended questionnaires with 10 mothers and three fathers, as well as with one of the founders of IPeP. We asked how parents and professionals negotiate parenthood in times of the COVID crisis and in the face of (over)intensifying parenting ideologies (Güney-Frahm, 2020). In addition, a selection of Dutch Islamic parenting blogs/sites were analysed through participatory (digital) ethnography combining content analysis of social media data and interviews (with bloggers and followers).

Several of our interviewees stated they were astonished by the massive amount of communication and the instant responses of parents around them. One mother said that the WhatsApp message group 'exploded' with parents asking for worksheets. She said that the school had to intervene by emailing parents that pre-schoolers should not be bothered with school tasks for many continuous hours. Anxiety in relation to school(work) surfaced in several interviews. According to our participants, parent WhatsApp groups are known for their information overload and are perceived as arenas for 'parent shaming', with the 'parent entrepreneur' as the benchmark against which all deviations are measured. Several interviewees stated that most parents did not (dare to) share their struggles in managing (the balance in) home schooling, work and housekeeping. Some interviewees, however, seemed to resist parental anxiety by referring to their own (migration) background:

> My parents were guest workers [...] so I'm not used to parents interfering with your school or getting help with your homework [...] And when I look at my children, they have it all. What are we talking about?

As parents were becoming 'full-time professional teachers', according to some interviewees, we came across many self-manufactured day schedules on social media sites. Blogger Fatima, for instance, shared a schedule entitled 'The-holiday-that-isn't-a-holiday'. It contains a rather detailed description of the day, which is arranged in timeslots like 'learning time', 'creativity time' (drawing, modelling with clay, painting, writing) and 'religious time' (Qur'an reading or repetitive prayer). Interestingly, most online followers responded positively to these daily schedules, stating that these work well for them. We came across just a few critical remarks, such as people asking whether parents could 'also just go outdoors with their children, like going for a walk or cycling?'. However, in interviews, there were only a few positive appraisals of these schedules; for example, when interviewees applauded them as ways to meet the (developmental) needs of their children. Most interviewees – whom we spoke with one or two weeks after the peak – were inclined to criticise the day schedules as unfeasible and not meeting the needs of children and (working) parents. The time lag may be one explanation: like us, as scholar-parents, they may have also grown increasingly intolerant of the detailed orchestration of daily life. On the other hand, it is also likely that parents felt more at ease in private communication to disqualify the (intensive-parenting-like) shaming of parents who fail to manage their child (and their school life).

The day schedule and the act of sharing it on social media square with intensive parenting discourse. It shows the internalisation of notions like self-management and child-centredness (Hays, 1996). All schedules were designed and applied by parents (and children) themselves. The way they resembled school days on the one hand, but included timeslots for creativity, relaxing and religious education on the other, shows a professionalised take on the parenting 'job'. No one mentions teachers or mosques facilitating parents in organising their day proactively. Not a single schedule we encountered included a timeslot for parents' work or free time. Most interviewees said they had to prioritise home schooling over their job, which forced parents to work evenings and weekends. Parents' instant reaction to school closure of assigning themselves a professional educational role has led us to speak of a 'self-responsibilisation reflex'.

Pivotal moments: intensive parenting destabilised?

The COVID crisis, however, may very well prove to be a pivotal moment. In quarantine, parents have been heard shouting from the (digital) rooftops: parenting is too absorbing, too expensive, too child-centred, too expert-driven, too individualistic, too unequal, too intense! The Muslim parents we encountered online, for instance, used the digital spaces of organisations like IPeP and Kleine Moslims to discuss and reconsider the way in which 'good parenting' is often defined according to intensive parenting standards of educational support, that is, parental involvement in the academic progress and extracurricular activities of children. Parents who do not (overtly) portray intense engagement are likely to be accused of doing a poor job of managing school–parent interaction (Din, 2017). In our COVID dataset, such accusations occurred; there were also question marks with respect to the intensity of school life at home and the responsibility of parents in this regard.

That this might be a pivotal moment is evident in the following data. Dutch Muslim Instagram mommy blogger 'Fatimama' (17 March 2020) initially seems to be the epitome of the intensified self-responsibilisation:

> Due to the large supply [of educational materials] I feel the pressure to continually offer them something educational. So I asked N's teacher if the school assignments were enough … I have stress about a lot of things but the schools are closed … Teacher Tanya responds: 'Perfect! Make the most of your quality time … Do something fun together and enjoy it!'
>
> *(Fatimama, 17 March 2020)*

However, her positioning shifted three days later, when she stated that the educational support she needs to provide ought to be limited. She explicitly detaches herself from the double role she was assigned and had briefly appropriated:

> I'm not a teacher now. They already have one. I'm a mother and I have to take care we don't bash each other's brains in.
>
> *(Fatimama, 20 March 2020)*

It is interesting to see Fatimama presenting this detachment as an autonomous decision, completely omitting the reassuring message from teacher Tanya. In various interviews, comparable pivotal moments surfaced. Parents reflect on how, after a while, they 'came to their senses', arguing that their educational endeavours turned out to be unfeasible, too demanding and not meeting their child's needs. Attention was redirected to connectedness and closeness to their children. Although such turns away from 'parents-as-teachers-and-family managers' were not directly visible on the social media sites that we studied, we did observe a change of tone, emphasising children's play and a more personal, small-context approach.

Intensive parenting with an Islamic inflection?

Notwithstanding experiences of exhaustion and work–family life imbalance during the first weeks of lockdown, most parents emphasised they have cherished family quality time, although this could be interpreted as a perpetuation of the 'feeling rules' of (online) parenting culture (Pedersen and Lupton, 2018). Parents also believed that the lockdown situation spurred spiritual enrichment in their families. Both online and offline, we came across parents who claimed to prepare more consciously for the holy month Ramadan, spend more time on religious education, work on their intentions (*niyyah*) and appreciate religious obligations as favours that can easily be taken away. Several interviewees said that it was easier to practise and nurture their faith: no more awkwardness about not shaking hands or (Christian) feasts at school.

Similarly, chaplain Hamza Akkar, one of the editors of Facebook page IPeP, refers to the concept of *al-qadar* (divine fate) in his webinar Islamic Emotion Regulation: Corona. This concept pertains to the notion that all disasters that strike the earth are already registered by Allah (Qur'an 57:22). Islamic (spi)ritual practices, like prayer (*salat*), are put forward as important cures for COVID. Relying on God's will should make believers all but passive or fatalistic; as Akkar explains, *al-qadar* also indicates that God created mankind with free will and responsibility. In his webinar, Akkar brings across a message of spiritual trust and relatedness to both Allah and the community of believers ('*ummah*').

The believer's responsibility was addressed in several questions asked by participants at the webinar. For some, this seemed to result in the religious version of the earlier mentioned self-responsibilisation reflex. One participant asked Akkar: 'Have I fallen short as a parent when my children do not pray correctly?'. Although Akkar nuances this self-reproach by stating that perhaps circumstances might play a role and that 'you could see it as an opportunity to improve', the notion of exclusive responsibility of parents and the presupposed (uni-)causal effect of their deeds remain underlined, seemingly turning a sacred *responsibility* into sacred *responsibilisation*. The topic briefly touched the surface on IPeP's Facebook page some weeks later, where a follower states that 'it takes a village to raise children', in the context of a discussion on how to teach children to pray.

These ambivalent stances on individualised (religious) parenting contrast with the very existence and mission statements of Islamic parenting support sites like that of IPeP, which are often grounded in notions of solidarity within the Muslim community (Islamic Pedagogy and Psychology Practices, 2020). Very much in line with the thought that 'it takes a village', Islamic parenting is here considered to be an inherently communal effort.

NIDA, racism and the COVID outbreak

Study 2 exposed cracks *outside* the family domain, where political organisations such as NIDA make a public case against racism and take over responsibilities to fight racism and become resilient in the face of it from individual families. In the Netherlands, open discussion of sociopolitical issues such as coronavirus-related racism seems to be completely off the public agenda. Unfortunately, Islamophobic ideas and practices still roam freely in Dutch society (Essed and Hoving, 2015), politics (Mutsaers et al., 2014) and institutions (e.g. Mutsaers, 2019a), developments that are known for their detrimental effects on families (Miller and Vittrup, 2020). In line with doctrines of 'parenting pedagogies' and the 'parent-citizen' (Edwards et al., 2013), intensive parenting allocates racism and stigmatisation as problems to be solved within the family domain, where family members ought to become resilient and should overcome racism through self-management and proper cultivation. As mentioned above, intensive parenting ideology prefers to target the 'parent-citizen' in this regard (Edwards et al., 2013). In this section, we turn to racialisation and Islamophobia in pandemic times and the positioning of NIDA in the racism debate.

As indicated above, several interviewees considered the COVID outbreak an opportunity for spiritual enrichment, but some of them also criticised the Dutch government's response to COVID-related racism. One interviewee, for instance, posted a remark on the Dutch media framing of Muslims during the pandemic and how it may indicate institutionalised discrimination. This interviewee had even tried to contact the media several times in the past before deciding it was useless.

As we mentioned in the introduction, the current generation of Dutch Muslim parents is pioneering by actively and publicly confronting stigmatisation and polarisation. Embodying these developments in the political arena, NIDA is actively championing cultural and religious diversity (Valenta, 2015). Fighting racism and Islamophobia plays an important role in that regard (NIDA, 2020). Public and academic debates on Islamophobia are continuing, but it can be argued that Muslims have been the object of racialisation throughout (Dutch) history (De Koning, 2016). To NIDA, racism and Islamophobia are part and parcel of the same discriminatory climate in the Netherlands. Going against the grain of such individualisation and (self)-responsibilisation, NIDA's efforts in these pandemic times can be interpreted, we argue, as a continuation of an emancipatory movement that was already set in motion for the benefit of second- and third-generation Muslims (Slootman, 2017).

Public pedagogy with an Islamic inflection

Months before the worldwide anti-racism protests (triggered by the death of the American George Floyd in May 2020) had begun in earnest and the streets of Dutch cities were engulfed by protesters, NIDA had already started to connect issues of racism, Islamophobia and the coronavirus. Founded on the idea that Muslim communities were not being heard enough in Dutch politics, NIDA describes itself as an emancipation movement inspired by Islam; its members are often actively involved in debates on religious and cultural diversity, in particular concerning Dutch Muslims and their position in society. Such debates tend to concern 'internal' affairs (for example, during the COVID pandemic, an exchange of ideas was stimulated by how to deal with Islamic burials and the rituals involved), but attention is also directed to the varied inequities that Muslims face in the Netherlands, especially during challenging times such as public health crises. NIDA's current leader Nourdin el Ouali has an educational background in pedagogy. El Ouali's interventions in debates on, for example, parenting styles in Moroccan-Dutch families (Samuel, 2018), are an illustration of NIDA's positioning as a pedagogical-political movement that stands up for Islamic communities in the Netherlands. El Ouali's public pedagogy can be juxtaposed with intensive parenting's privatisation of racism (or Islamophobia, for that matter); he and the party persevere in redirecting attention to Dutch society and how it can be 'educated' for the sake of inclusion and diversity.

As we know, pandemics and concomitant public health debates often add grist to the racist mill, and ensuing discourses may outlast the pandemic (Briggs, 2005). It is therefore unsurprising that NIDA was quick to respond to the first signs of Islamophobia in the media. However, as El Ouali has explicitly expressed during this pandemic, for NIDA the outbreak also provides an opportunity to further draw attention to the shortcomings of government and society in general. By doing that, NIDA is also challenging ideologies of the intensive parenting system by working out a public pedagogy (i.e. through their social activism). As such, our interviewees, who have objected to forms of corona racism, are acknowledged and supported by the social activism NIDA engages in for the benefit of Dutch Muslim communities.

'Did you notice this too?'

In this final section, we briefly discuss a case study of a particular form of social activism in which NIDA engages: its criticism of media framing of Muslims during the COVID outbreak. About a week before the Dutch government announced strict measures in response to the pandemic, NIDA posted a video on its Facebook page that focused on the representation of Muslim women in media coverage of the pandemic. A story, posted shortly before the video, was given the title *Was dit jou ook opgevallen?* ('Did you notice this too?'). In the video, we see El Ouali engaged in a conversation with several of his fellow party members and calling on newspaper offices to question editorial boards about mediatised photos of veiled Muslim women in articles about COVID. Such framing was not only noticed by political parties such as DENK (national) and NIDA (local), which both give a voice to Dutch Muslims, but also by a number of public commentators (e.g. Slaats, 2020) and on social media.

Media representation of Muslims has been a long-standing concern (e.g. Morey and Yaqin, 2011), but not in the context of pandemics. According to Briggs, however, pandemics can easily be racialised, since

> middle-class, heterosexual whites are seldom stigmatised by diseases, but racialised and/or sexualised populations become marked in ways that can long

> outlive the epidemic. As media feeding frenzies retell narratives, visual images powerfully link racialised bodies with descriptions of disease.
>
> *(Briggs, 2005: 276)*

In this particular case, the link was established between Muslim women (a continuous 'object' of racialisation and sexualisation in Western media) and the spreading of a new virus. Such ideology must be viewed as a 'privileged silence' most effectively entrenched when achieving the status of 'common sense' (Fairclough, 1992). In this case, all media representatives contacted by NIDA seemed to be oblivious to any kind of intentional framing. When asked about the photo selection, a representative of a popular daily (*Metro*) responded: 'I wouldn't know. I did not notice this'. Others responded agitatedly: 'The picture that you paint is just not correct. I really think that you are looking for things that aren't there. I think we should not exaggerate things'. A spokesperson for the *Algemeen Dagblad* seems exasperated when asked if there was any 'sensitivity' in selecting this particular photo: 'What do you mean, sensitivity? I feel a little despondent about all this. I really don't have time for these sort of reflections.'

This NIDA action brought to the surface what otherwise would have remained invisible and unnoticed. It provided an opportunity for such media coverage to be drained of political potency, and it gave the message, once again, that Muslims in the Netherlands are a community not to be reckoned with. By suggesting that the link between COVID and Muslim women in this form of framing is not unintentional (regardless of what media representatives themselves say about it), NIDA gives weight to the idea that racism is exacerbated in pandemic times, whether through governmental attitudes or mass media. Similarly, several interviewees criticised the Dutch prime minister's latest Ramadan message ('Stay at home!'), that – contrasting with his Easter message – resonated a tone of suspicion specifically directed at Dutch Muslims, linking this to his earlier problematic statements and attitudes towards Islam in Dutch society. We suggest that such examples demonstrate forms of resistance to what Briggs (2005: 277–279) refers to as 'geographies of blame', in which institutionalised cultural stereotypes are employed to link diseases to racialised minorities.

Finally, it should be noted that the Facebook clip, which garnered considerable attention, as evidenced in the comments, emoticons and sharing it yielded, gives the impression of a (NIDA) family whose members are there to look after each other. This counter-narrative connects seamlessly with NIDA's self-presentation and public pedagogy of extended family structures as foundational to social cohesion and parenting as a 'common good'. The importance of family in NIDA's view can be found on both the level of the Muslim communities that they represent and embody, and on the level of the whole of society and its well-functioning, to which family life is foundational. Discrimination, in this case in the form of COVID-related racism, disrupts this foundation (NIDA, 2020).

Conclusion

In this chapter, we explored how a dominant ideology of intensive parenting can be seen at work in the guise of (self-)responsibilisation. Considering the 'reflexes' we encountered, intensive parenting can indeed be seen as an effective ideology, with its logics being internalised and thereby normalised. On the other hand, the COVID crisis also appears to have caused or exposed small 'cracks in the system'. Some (but not all) parents seem to resist the responsibility for educational support that is transferred onto their shoulders. This can be seen as a reaction to the 'self-responsibilisation reflex' they have seen around them or which they have found themselves doing. The intensification of parent–school relations, which has led to a blending of private and public spheres (a 'context collapse') is experienced as too far-reaching. Perhaps, the lockdown has made things so invasive that parents now reconsider and reinterpret the dominant role that school is playing in their families' lives. In any case, for some parents, their migration background enabled them to detach themselves from hegemonic norms prioritising nuclear family structures. We saw more ambivalent stances regarding religious responsibilities of parents, which might have to do with the theological importance of this topic. Yet, the 'cracks' that these parents experienced seemed to redirect them towards reflection and connectedness, both familial and spiritual.

We have observed similar cracks in NIDA's dealings with COVID-related racism. Reminiscent of the older works of critical pedagogues such as Henry A. Giroux and Peter McLaren (e.g. Giroux and McLaren, 1989), NIDA is continuing its ongoing efforts to 'educate society' rather than merely the individuals it contains. Such a 'public pedagogy' stands in stark contrast to the singular focus on individual (family) members that is prioritised in intensive parenting ideology. Rather than abiding to the ideal of (self-)responsibilisation and individual resilience, NIDA sweeps the discussion back to the public domain, effectively acting out a public pedagogy. Although giving attention to the public rather than the private, the collective rather than the individual, the structural rather than the incidental is not unique (it is arguably the very core of anti-racist movements; Mutsaers, 2019b) it may be more important than ever before, now that we live in times of locked-down individuals and quarantined families.

Acknowledgements

We thank Ernst van den Hemel, Herman Beck and Yoeri van Helvoirt for their perceptive, helpful comments on an earlier draft of this chapter, and Yasmina Yusuf and Alexander den Toom for their contribution to our fieldwork. A special thanks goes out to the editors of this book, Deborah Lupton and Karen Willis, for their thorough editing job. This study is financed by the Dutch Research Council (NWO).

References

Blommaert J (2005) *Discourse*. Cambridge: Cambridge University Press.

Briggs CL (2005) Communicability, racial discourse, and disease. *Annual Review of Anthropology* 34: 269–291.

De Koning M (2016) 'You need to present a counter-message': the racialisation of Dutch Muslims and anti-Islamophobia initiatives. *Journal of Muslims in Europe* 5: 170–189.

Din S (2017) *Muslim Mothers and their Children's Schooling*. London: Trentham Books.

Edwards V, Gillies G and Horsely E (2013) *Challenging the Politics of Early Intervention: Who's 'Saving' Children and Why*. Bristol: Policy Press.

Essed P and Hoving I (eds) (2015) *Dutch Racism*. Leiden: Brill.

Faircloth C and Murray M (2015) Parenting: kinship, expertise, and anxiety. *Journal of Family Issues* 36 (9): 1115–1129.

Fairclough N (1992) *Discourse and Social Change*. Cambridge: Polity.

Geigner F, Vandenbroek M and Roets G (2014) Parenting as a performance: parents as consumers and (de)constructors of mythic parenting and childhood ideals. *Childhood* 21 (4): 488–501.

Giroux HA and McLaren P (1989) *Critical Pedagogy, the State and Cultural Struggle*. Albany, NY: State University of New York Press.

Güney-Frahm I (2020) Neoliberal motherhood during the pandemic: some reflections. *Gender, Work & Organization* 27 (5): 847–856.

Hall S (1985) Signification, representation, ideology: Althusser and the post-structuralist debates. *Critical Studies in Media Communication* 2 (2): 91–114.

Hays S (1996) *The Cultural Contradictions of Motherhood*. New Haven, CT: Yale University Press.

Islamic Pedagogy and Psychology Practices (2020) Hoe versterk ik mijn zelfbeeld en dat van mijn kind? Retrieved from https://ipepacademy.nl/islamzelfbeeld (accessed 18 June 2020).

Maliepaard M and Alba R (2016) Cultural integration in the Muslim second generation in the Netherlands: the case of gender ideology. *International Migration Review* 50 (1): 70–94.

Miller C and Vittrup B (2020) The indirect effects of police racial bias on African American families. *Journal of Family Issues* 41 (10): 1699–1722.

Morey P and Yaqin A (2011) *Framing Muslims*. Cambridge, MA: Harvard University Press.

Mutsaers P, Siebers H, and de Ruijter A (2014) Becoming a minority: ethno-manufacturing in the Netherlands. In: Tripathy J and Padmanabhan S (eds) *Becoming Minority: How Discourses and Policies Produce Minorities in Europe and India*. Los Angeles, CA: Sage, pp. 174–195.

NIDA (2020) NIDA's Keuringsdienst van Waarde #corona #hoofddoek #mondkapje. Retrieved from www.facebook.com/NIDAfb/videos/575357803072823 (accessed 1 July 2020).

Ochs E and Kremer-Sadlik T (2015) How postindustrial families talk. *Annual Review of Anthropology* 44: 87–103.

Pang B (2020) Beyond hypervisibility and fear: British Chinese communities' leisure and health related experiences in the time of coronavirus. *Leisure Sciences*. Epub ahead of print.

Pedersen S and Lupton D (2018) 'What are you feeling right now?' communities of maternal feeling on Mumsnet. *Emotion, Space and Society* 26 (February): 57–63.

Pels T and de Gruijter M (2006) *Emancipatie van de tweede generatie: Keuzen en kansen in de levensloop van jonge moeders van Marokkaanse en Turkse afkomst*. Report. Utrecht: Verwey-Jonker Instituut.

Rezai S (2017) *The rise of the second generation: the role of social capital in the upward* mobility of descendants of immigrants from Turkey and Morocco. PhD thesis, Erasmus University Rotterdam, the Netherlands.

Rollock N, Gillborn D, Vincent C and Ball SJ (2014) *The Colour of Class: The Educational Strategies of the Black Middle Class*. London: Routledge.

Samuel M (2018) De Hervormingsfundamentalisten: Nourdin El Ouali 'Neem je eigenwaarde in eigen beheer'. Retrieved from www.mounirsamuel.nl/hervormingsfundamentalisten-nourdin-el-ouali-neem-eigenwaarde-eigen-beheer (accessed 16 June 2020).

Schenkels A and Mutsaers P (2019) *Intensive Islamic parenting in neoliberal times?* Canadian Anthropology Society and American Anthropologist Association Conference 'Changing Climates', Vancouver, Canada, 20–24 November.

Slaats J (2020) Corona en racisme: een beschamend facet van de pandemie. Retrieved from https://kifkif.be/cnt/artikel/corona-en-racisme-een-beschamend-facet-van-de-pandemie-8828 (accessed 16 June 2020).

Slootman M (2017) Social mobility allowing for ethnic identification: reassertion of ethnicity among Moroccan and Turkish Dutch. *International Migration* 56 (4): 125–139.

Valenta M (2015) Het voorbeeld van NIDA: Een veelbelovende emancipatiepartij nieuwe stijl. In: Buijs G and ten Hooven M (eds) *Nuchtere betogen over religie. Waarheid en verdichting over de publieke rol van godsdiensten.* Eindhoven: Damon, pp. 203–214.

16

ANTI-ASIAN RACISM, XENOPHOBIA AND ASIAN AMERICAN HEALTH DURING COVID-19

Aggie J. Yellow Horse

Introduction

The first confirmed case of COVID-19 in the US, on 19 January 2020, was a Chinese American in Washington who recently had returned from travelling to the Chinese city of Wuhan to visit family (Holshue et al., 2020). Although subsequent research has challenged the theory that Wuhan was the initial source of the COVID pandemic (Huang et al., 2020), anti-Asian racism and xenophobic rhetoric, as well as reports of hate incidents against Asian Americans, began to rise (Jeung et al., 2020). STOP AAPI HATE, a research–community partnership between Asian American Studies at San Francisco State, the Asian Pacific Policy and Planning Council (A3PCON) and Chinese for Affirmative Action (CAA), began to collect self-reported hate incidences against Asian Americans in mid-March and documented over 2,000 reports of hate incidents in just the first 10 weeks. Asian Americans have reported multiple forms of discrimination (e.g. verbal harassment, physical assaults, being spat on) at multiple spaces (e.g. private residence, public space, online) (Borja et al., 2020).

Understanding how such racist and xenophobic incidences may affect Asian Americans' physical, mental and social health is critical, as racism is the *fundamental* cause of health inequalities across social groups in the US (Phelan and Link, 2015; Paradies et al., 2015) and for Asian Americans (Gee, 2008). Such understanding is important for reducing and eliminating the barriers for Asian Americans seeking medical help during the coronavirus pandemic, as fear of experiencing hate incidents can deter individuals from seeking proper testing and care; and greatly affect Asian Americans' health. Furthermore, it also affects the health of the total US population, as the success of combating SARS-CoV-2 requires cooperation from everyone to succeed. Thus far, research about the health implications of the social, cultural and political dimensions of the coronavirus pandemic on Asian Americans is limited, due to pre-existing conceptual and methodological challenges in studying health and health inequities among Asian Americans. While it is important to document and investigate the rise in anti-Asian racism and xenophobia during COVID, I argue that examination of how they affect Asian American health must be situated within contexts critically examining the history of systemic marginalisation of Asian Americans in public health discourse.

In this chapter, I first discuss how COVID exacerbated racism and xenophobia against Asian Americans in the US. In doing so, I discuss the challenges of studying the impacts of COVID on Asian Americans' health and communities, and how such challenges stem from both pre-existing conceptual and methodological challenges. In conclusion, I discuss the importance of long-lasting and abiding institutional support in examining the roles of racism and xenophobia on Asian Americans' health and elaborate on suggestions for future research and policy advocacy.

Anti-Asian racism and xenophobia exacerbated during COVID

Since 2000, Asian Americans have been the fastest-growing racial minority group in the US. From 11.9 million who reported themselves in 2000 as having either full or partial Asian heritage (Barnes and Bennett, 2002), the number of Asian Americans has nearly doubled to 22.9 million in 2018 (increased from 4.2 to 7.0 per cent of the total US population) (United States Census Bureau, 2020). The population growth of Asian Americans is expected to continue: it is projected that Asian Americans will constitute about 14 per cent of the total US population by 2065 (compared to 24 per cent of Hispanics and 13 per cent of African Americans) (Cohn, 2015). Due to emphasis on family reunification and the employment preferences of post-1965 immigrants, Asian Americans are a highly selected group for educational qualifications and occupations.

Asian Americans have been experiencing a great deal of both individual and structural racism even prior to COVID. The report *Discrimination in America* documents that about a quarter of Asian Americans reported experiencing institutional forms of racism (e.g. unequal pay or consideration for promotions, discrimination in housing); and about one-third of Asian Americans reported experiencing individual forms of discrimination (e.g. racial or ethnic slurs, negative or offensive assumptions and comments about their race and ethnicity) (McMurtry et al., 2019).

Since the outbreak and spread of COVID in the US, Asian Americans have been reporting multiple forms of discrimination. According to research from the Pew Research Center (one of the few surveys that have included a representative sample of Asian Americans), Asian Americans and Black Americans have experienced significant discrimination amid the COVID outbreak (Ruiz et al., 2020). Nearly 39 per cent of Asian Americans indicated that 'people acted as if they were uncomfortable around them' because of their race; 31 per cent of Asian Americans have been subjected to racial slurs or jokes; and 26 per cent of Asian Americans indicated that they feared the possibility of threat or physical attack. Given that this survey was only conducted in

English (and therefore did not include Asian-born Americans who are not fluent in English), these figures are likely to be an underestimation of how many Asian Americans have experienced discrimination. Furthermore, as previous research documenting discrimination often omits Asian Americans, it is challenging to discern whether and how the discrimination that Asian Americans experience amid the pandemic reflects any changes in magnitude and intensity.

Another grassroots research-community partnership effort, STOP AAPI HATE, documents the significant hate incidents towards Asian Americans. The reports of hate incidents spiked after President Trump first used the term 'China virus' to refer to the novel coronavirus in a tweet (Borja et al., 2020). Since then, these incidents have consistently been reported. During the first 13 weeks, there were 2,089 hate incidents towards Asian Americans reported on the STOP AAPI HATE website. Of these 2,089 cases, multiple forms of hate incidents were reported, including verbal harassment and name-calling, shunning, physical assault, being coughed/spat on, online abuse, workplace discrimination and being barred from establishments and transportation. Asian Americans also suspected a variety of reasons for their experiences of discrimination, including race, ethnicity, wearing a mask, gender, language, food, religion, and others.

A special issue of *Journal of Asian American Studies*, organised to amplify the experiences of the lives of those perceived to be Asian, Asian American and/or Pacific Islander during COVID, documents how COVID has affected Asian Americans during the early phase of the pandemic (Yellow Horse et al., in press 2020). The collection show how intensively COVID impacted every part of the Asian American community, including, but not limited to, Asian American college students and academic staff, Asian Americans serving community-based organisations, and Asian American businesses across the US.

Taken together, these accounts clearly document the substantial experiences of racism and xenophobia towards Asian Americans during the COVID crisis. Yet research on assessing its impacts on Asian American health is still largely limited, due to conceptual and methodological issues. The COVID health paradox for Asian Americans is that despite substantial anti-Asian racism and xenophobia, COVID in *aggregate* measures does not seem to affect Asian Americans as much as other non-white groups. This false paradox narrative is heavily influenced by pre-existing conceptual and methodological issues, and exacerbates lack of knowledge about the health impacts of COVID on Asian American communities.

The conceptual challenges: the invisibility of Asian Americans in health research

Asian Americans have been rendered invisible in public health discourse from two seemingly contrasting racialised stereotypes of Asian Americans as model minorities and perpetual foreigners. These racialised stereotypes together enforce the oppression and marginalisation of Asian Americans. They operate to deny this group's unmet health needs and desires, including their access to health resources. As a 'model minority' with apparently relatively lower COVID infection rates, anti-Asian racism does not connect very intuitively to the difficulties of research with the Asian American communities in relation to COVID without understanding various historical contexts.

Asian Americans are comprised of individuals and their descendants from more than two dozen countries with unique immigration histories, cultures, modes of entry and policy contexts; yet they have become ascribed as a pan-ethnic group through racialisation and racial group formation (Espiritu, 1993; Omi and Winant, 1994). While the development of Asian American pan-ethnicity also reflects the achieved self-identity by Asian ethnic groups based on collective struggles as a political social movement symbol during the Civil Rights era (Espiritu, 1993; Zia, 2000), such collective identity is too often misunderstood as a signal of declining ethnic distinctions (Okamoto, 2014). In fact, many Americans have accepted the misconstrued notion of Asian American as a monolithic racial category in which Asian ethnic groups are forcefully confined into racial groupings. This in turn legitimises the misconception of homogeneity within Asian Americans (Hollinger, 2000). Although the pan-ethnicity as Asian Americans provided the tool for collective actions (Okamoto, 2003), it has also been misused to construct the model minority stereotype, where Asian Americans are reimagined as a homogenous racial group with socioeconomic success, upper mobility and overall wellbeing. The model minority myth conceals the deleterious health effects of historically institutional racism on Asian Americans, denies the health needs and desires of Asian Americans and obscures the heterogeneous health status of Asian American subgroups.

At a glance, the health profiles of Asian Americans *overall* appear to fit well the 'model minority myth', as Asian Americans typically appear to have better health profiles than the general US population. Asian Americans have the longest life expectancy compared to other racial and ethnic groups (Acciai et al., 2015), a higher proportion self-reporting 'good' health status and a lower prevalence of physical chronic conditions in general (Bloom and Black, 2016). However, the data disaggregation by countries of origin among Asian Americans quickly unravels the stark health inequities within Asian Americans (Bloom and Black, 2016). Health profiles of Asian Americans are further complicated by the relative health advantages of foreign-born Asian Americans (John et al., 2012).

In addition, it is important to acknowledge that health inequities can exist in the absence of observed differences in health indicators, based on how individuals perceive and feel about their own health. For example, if we interpret having access to health insurance coverage as an indicator of 'good health' status for Asian Americans, it could lead to the assumption that there are no health inequities among Asian Americans. Yet, Asian Americans may have qualitatively distinct perceptions of what 'good health' means (for example, having the freedom or time to seek healthcare). It also masks the need to systematically integrate the role of anti-Asian racism and xenophobia into understanding the health inequities of Asian Americans.

Despite the presence and contributions of Asian Americans since the middle of the 19th century (Takaki, 1990), Asian Americans are simultaneously reimagined as the 'perpetual foreigners' who are unable or unwilling to acculturate to dominant US values because of racist nativism. The perpetual foreigner stereotype is built on hysteria about Asian Americans that is deeply rooted in anti-East Asian racism originating from the Yellow Peril xenophobic ideology in the mid-19th century, where Asians were viewed as a threat to the Western world (Lyman, 2000). At this time, many Americans felt threatened by an increase in immigration from China on the basis of labour tensions and shifting national identities. Racist, patriarchal and capitalist institutions have long used Asian Americans as scapegoats by associating diseases with 'foreigners' and shaped the meanings of race and citizenship through public health concerns (Shah, 2001; Molina, 2006; Lee, 2019).

Furthermore, a series of racist legislations was instituted to halt immigration from Asia. Asian Americans are the first and only group in the US to have been legally banned from immigration through a series of discriminatory legislations based on race. These regulations included, for example, the Chinese Exclusion Act of 1882, the Gentlemen's Agreement of 1907, and the Immigration Act of 1924. Such race-based discriminatory exclusion of Asian Americans did not cease until the immigration ban based on race and quota was lifted with introduction of the Immigration Act of 1965. Conceptualising Asian Americans as perpetual foreigners, Americans will likely continue to hold a restrictionist view (that is, anti-Asian racist nativism) which not only symbolically denies societal membership granting access to health resources but positions Asian Americans as 'other'.

Through these racialised stereotypes, Asian Americans are either imagined as the group who is doing well (thus ignoring the need to examine the role of anti-racism and xenophobia) or as the outsiders who are not an integral part of the mitigating efforts for the total US population. Furthermore, such racialisation influences Asian Americans' health behaviours. For example, some Asian Americans may choose to not wear a mask to avoid the increased probability of experiencing hate incidents (that is, fear of being assumed as infected or bringing infection as the perpetual foreigner). Simultaneously, mask wearing contributes to the model minority discourse as not showing independence and freedom, hence less American.

The methodological challenges in data collection

It has been hard to obtain accurate and reliable basic data assessing the true effects of COVID for Asian Americans, due to the lack of Asian American representation in COVID data. Given the relatively small population size of Asian Americans by ethnic origin, it is important to consider carefully the geographic scale for data release to protect the anonymity of individuals. However, reliable and accurate COVID statistics for Asian American subgroups at the aggregate level are critical to an accurate estimation of the pandemic's impacts on Asian Americans. For example, in San Francisco, one of the places with high percentages of Asian Americans; Asian Americans account for nearly half of COVID deaths and the Asian American case fatality rate is four times higher compared to the overall population (Yan et al., 2020). However, at a larger aggregate level, such as the state, Asian Americans' disproportionate experiences of COVID are masked. Unfortunately, this challenge is not new.

Asian Americans have been rendered invisible in public health discourse due to methodological challenges as well. That is, they are often excluded in race-based health statistics by either being completely omitted or lumped into the 'other' category with other racial and ethnic groups. When Asian Americans are included, they are often misrepresented as a monolithic pan-ethnic group without highlighting the important group differences, or simply used as a comparison group (Holland and Palaniappan, 2012). Explanations for such exclusion are often grounded in two 'methodological' challenges specific to data collection: first, Asian Americans constitute a small proportion of the US total population; and second, the heterogeneity of Asian Americans adds another layer of complexity to data collection.

The first methodological challenge is grounded in the argument that as a small proportion of the total population the current health profiles and needs of Asian Americans cannot be generalisable to the total population, and thus have less public health significance. For example, many nationally representative surveys only include either the pan-ethnic category of Asian Americans or a few selected Asian American subgroups. These surveys only recently began to oversample Asian Americans; for example, the National Health and Nutrition Examination Survey began oversampling Asian Americans in 2011 (Paulose-Ram et al., 2017).

The second methodological challenge is that substantial heterogeneity within Asian Americans creates barriers for collecting a robust representative sample of Asian Americans. The 1965 Immigration and Naturalization Act, which removed national quotas set in place in 1924, resulted in the rapid increase of Asian migration to the US. The 1965 legislation instituted categories based on skilled and unskilled labour, family reunification, and refugee states (Hing, 1993). As a result, some Asian Americans entering the United States have entered under H1B visas for in-demand, highly skilled labour or with EB-5 visas (created in 1990) for entrepreneurs, or less skilled and less wealthy and entering by virtue of family reunification (or chain migration) policies. The new streams of Asian immigrants contribute to the heterogeneity. The large number of foreign-born Asian Americans adds complexities, such as differences in nativity, language, citizenship status, generational status and acculturation (Srinivasan and Guillermo, 2000).

Based on these two methodological challenges, most nationally representative survey data has a small and underrepresented sample of Asian Americans because of inadequate sampling coverage, selection and non-response (Lee and Baik, 2011), preventing researchers from disaggregating Asian Americans to investigate the within-group differences among Asian Americans by ethnicity (Ward and Byrd, 2012; Walton, 2009; Lee and Baik, 2011). However, adequate Asian American representation in data and explicit investigation of within-group ethnic differences among Asian Americans are important both theoretically and empirically. Ethnicity is a complex two-dimensional social construct that is central to health inequalities:

it defines both group characteristics and a group's relational location within a social hierarchy (Ford and Harawa, 2010). Methodologically, combining distinct ethnic groups leads to erroneous conclusions that mask the critical heterogeneity between and within various ethnic groups (Uehara et al., 1994).

This argument for the critical need of adequate representation data is not new (Srinivasan and Guillermo, 2000) nor specific to only Asian Americans (e.g. lack of Indigenous representation in data). Such 'methodological' challenges are rooted in long-standing anti-Asian racism and what is legible to policy-makers; and public health researchers and policy-makers must continue to examine the role of institutional racism in the continual lack of representation of Asian Americans in public health data.

To increase Asian American representation in this data, there have been several important forefront national data collection efforts organised by leading Asian American scholar-activists, including but not limited to: the 2002–2003 National Latino and Asian American Study (Alegria and Takeuchi, 2003), the 2008 and 2016 National Asian American Surveys (Ramakrishnan et al., 2008; Ramakrishnan et al., 2016), and the 2008 and 2016 Collaborative Multiracial Post-election Surveys (Barreto et al., 2017; Barreto et al., 2008). These data collection efforts make it possible for researchers to ask time-relevant and nuanced questions that are important to Asian American families and communities.

Conclusion: assessing the effects of racism, xenophobia and Asian American health

The need to accurately and reliably assess the impacts of COVID on Asian Americans' health is imperative – especially with added stressors like experiences of increased racism and xenophobia; yet pre-existing conceptual and methodological challenges in understanding Asian Americans' health conjointly contributes to inadequate representation of Asian Americans in health research during COVID. The COVID crisis has brought multiple questions and challenges for public health researchers and policy-makers for advocating for health equities of Asian Americans.

First, the rapid increase in incidences of racist and xenophobic hate towards Asian Americans has brought the importance of *explicitly* including systemic racism and discrimination as a fundamental cause of the health inequities Asian Americans experience. Despite disturbingly being an ascribed 'model minority' who supposedly have achieved tremendous economic success through hard work and family values, the rapid increase in incidences of racist and xenophobic hate towards Asian Americans during the pandemic showed that Asian Americans are not immune to racism and discrimination. Specifically, the need to systematically investigate how racism and xenophobia conjointly affect Asian Americans' health became clear. For example, Asian Americans who work in healthcare report substantial numbers of hate incidences while working to combat the spread of the coronavirus (Kaiser Health News, 2020). Understanding racism as the fundamental cause of health inequalities (Link and Phelan, 1995) affecting individuals' health through multiple interconnected mechanisms means that the association between racism and health inequities and inequalities would persist even after controlling for other risk factors. Adequately addressing the role of systematic racism in understanding health inequities for Asian Americans is important because (1) an individual-centred approach to health inequities inaccurately puts the responsibilities and causes of inequities on individuals without accounting for the social contexts, and (2) policy solutions should be designed that address the racism directly rather than mechanisms (Cogburn, 2019; Hicken et al., 2018).

Second, there needs to be greater institutional support dedicated to more nuanced approaches to how we measure racism and discrimination for Asian Americans, and how multiple reasons for discrimination simultaneously occur to interact with one another. There is a clear need for a more intersectional approach to understanding Asian American experiences and health at the intersection of race, class, gender, immigration/citizenship status and place within a framework that acknowledges the social determinants of health (Collins, 1990). While Asian American psychologists and public health scholars paved the ways for investigating the health inequities of Asian Americans, especially with critical attention to the deleterious health effects of racism and discrimination within the social determinants of health framework (Hwang and Goto, 2008; Yoo et al., 2009; Liang et al., 2004; Alegria and Takeuchi, 2003), there are important complexities that future research needs to identify.

For Asian Americans, understanding the effects of racism on health is complicated by their unique position in racial stratification within racial triangulation theory (Kim, 1999), which suggests that racial stratification is multidimensional; that is, Asian Americans may be simultaneously rated high on one dimension and low on others.[1] Dr Claire Kim argues that Asian Americans are uniquely positioned in a 'field of racial positions' (Kim, 1999: 106) based on two axes: the *racial valorisation* process (i.e. racial hierarchy) and the *civic ostracism* process (i.e. insiders vs outsiders/foreigners) (Xu and Lee, 2013). This unique position poses additional questions for understanding the effects of racism on the health of Asian Americans: (1) how distinct ethnicities figure into racial triangulation when racial categories create the misleading aggregate; (2) whether and how the survey instruments developed to predominantly measure the experiences of racism and discrimination for Black Americans would be valid and effective in measuring the experiences of racism and discrimination for Asian Americans; (3) how to deconstruct the reasons for experiences of racism and discrimination, as Asian Americans can be discriminated against based on race or other indicators (for example, detangling racial from language discrimination) (Yoo et al., 2009).

Lastly, in addition to the explicit inclusion of racism and xenophobia in understanding Asian American health, the rapid response studies attempting to document the impacts of COVID on Asian American communities must oversample different ethnic groups of Asian Americans in order to make the data disaggregation possible, as the methodological challenges are rooted in long-standing anti-Asian racism. Furthermore, research should offer multiple Asian languages. In light of the lack of Asian American representation in the data, the limitations of quantitative inquiries in health research and the urgency of timely research communication during the COVID crisis, there is a need for researchers to work with communities and use multiple modes of inquiry to centre Asian Americans' experiences and health, such as participatory action research and community partnership. That is, it is not only important to systematically collect the data on Asian American experiences and changes in health during COVID, but researchers must also communicate the findings in formats that are readily accessible to the public (for example, policy briefs) and use such data to mobilise resources for the communities in return.

The COVID crisis has yet again exposed racism as a critical public health concern (Devakumar et al., 2020). As the COVID is ongoing and ever-shifting in nature, addressing elimination of the barriers to understanding the true impacts of COVID on Asian American health must be rooted in abiding and lasting systemic changes, in addition to rapid responses based on the history of systemic marginalisation of Asian Americans in public health discourse.

Note

1 For a thoughtful and nuanced yet succinct discussion of racial triangulation theory, racial formation theory, and the racial hierarchy/colour line(s) approach, see Xu and Lee (2013).

References

Acciai F, Noah AJ and Firebaugh G (2015) Pinpointing the sources of the Asian mortality advantage in the USA. *Journal of Epidemiology & Community Health* 69 (10): 1006–1011.

Alegria M and Takeuchi D (2003) National Latino and Asian American study. Retrieved from www.massgeneral.org/mongan-institute/centers/dru/research/past/nlaas (accessed 2 October 2020).

Barnes JS and Bennett CE (2002) *The Asian Population, 2000*. Washington, DC: US Department of Commerce, Economics and Statistics Administration.

Barreto M, Frasure-Yokley L, Vargas E and Wong J (2017) Collaborative multiracial post-election survey (CMPS), 2016. Retrieved from http://cmpsurvey.org/wp-content/uploads/2017/09/cmps_methodology.pdf (accessed 2 October 2020).

Barreto MA, Frasure-Yokley L, Hancock A-M, Manzano, S, Ramakrishnan SK, Ramirez R, Sancjhez G and Wong J (2008) Collaborative multi-racial post-election survey (CMPS), 2008. Inter-university Consortium for Political and Social Research (distributor). Retrieved from www.icpsr.umich.edu/web/RCMD/studies/35163/versions/V1 (accessed 2 October 2020).

Bloom B and Black LI (2016) Health of non-Hispanic Asian adults: United States, 2010–2014. *NCHS Data Brief* 247 (May): 1–8.

Borja M, Jeung R, Yellow Horse AJet al. (2020) China xenophobia tied to racism against Asian Americans. Retrieved from www.asianpacificpolicyandplanningcouncil.org/wp-content/uploads/Anti-China_Rhetoric_Report_6_17_20.pdf (accessed 2 October 2020).

Cogburn CD (2019) Culture, race, and health: implications for racial inequities and population health. *The Milbank Quarterly* 97 (3): 736–761.

Cohn D. (2015) Future immigration will change the face of America by 2065. Retrieved from www.pewresearch.org/fact-tank/2015/10/05/future-immigration-will-change-the-face-of-america-by-2065 (accessed 2 October 2020).

Collins PH (1990) *Black Feminist Thought: Knowledge, Consciousness, and the Politics of Empowerment*. New York: Routledge.

Devakumar D, Shannon G, Bhopal SSet al. (2020) Racism and discrimination in COVID-19 responses. *The Lancet* 395 (10231): 1194.

Espiritu YL (1993) *Asian American Panethnicity: Bridging Institutions and Identities*. Philadelphia, PA: Temple University Press.

Ford CL and Harawa NT (2010) A new conceptualization of ethnicity for social epidemiologic and health equity research. *Social Science & Medicine* 71: 251–258.

Gee GC (2008) A multilevel analysis of the relationship between institutional and individual racial discrimination and health status. *American Journal of Public Health* 98 (S1): 48–56.

Hicken MT, Kravitz-Wirtz N, Durkee M and Jackson JS (2018) Racial inequalities in health: framing future research. *Social Science & Medicine* 199: 11–18.

Hing BO (1993) *Making and Remaking Asian America through Immigration Policy: 1850–1990*. California: Stanford University Press.

Holland AT and Palaniappan LP (2012) Problems with the collection and interpretation of Asian-American health data: omission, aggregation, and extrapolation. *Annals of Epidemiology* 22 (6): 397–405.

Hollinger DA (2000) *Postethnic America: Beyond Multiculturalism*. New York: Basic Books.

Holshue ML, DeBolt C, Lindquist Set al. (2020) First case of 2019 novel coronavirus in the United States. *New England Journal of Medicine* 382: 929–936.

Huang C, Wang Y, Li Xet al. (2020) Clinical features of patients infected with 2019 novel coronavirus in Wuhan, China. *The Lancet* 395 (10223): 497–506.

Hwang W-C and Goto S (2008) The impact of perceived racial discrimination on the mental health of Asian American and Latino college students. *Cultural Diversity and Ethnic Minority Psychology* 14 (4): 326–335.

Jeung R, Gowing S and Takasaki K (2020) *News Accounts of COVID-19 Xenophobia: Types of Xenophobic Reactions, January 28–February 24, 2020*. Stop AAPI Hate Report. San Francisco, CA: Asian Pacific Policy & Planning Council (A3PCON) and Chinese for Affirmative Action (CAA).

John DA, De Castro A, Martin DP, Duran B and Takeuchi DT (2012) Does an immigrant health paradox exist among Asian Americans? Associations of nativity and occupational class with self-rated health and mental disorders. *Social Science & Medicine* 75: 2085–2098.

Kaiser Health News (2020) More verbal, physical attacks: Asian-American health care workers report rise in bigoted incidents. Retrieved from https://khn.org/morning-breakout/more-verbal-physical-attacks-asian-american-health-care-workers-report-rise-in-bigoted-incidents (accessed 2 October 2020).

Kim CJ (1999) The racial triangulation of Asian Americans. *Politics & Society* 27 (1): 105–138.

Lee E (2019) *America for Americans: A History of Xenophobia in the United States*. New York: Basic Books.

Lee H and Baik S-Y (2011) Health disparities or data disparities: sampling issues in hepatitis B Virus infection among Asian American Pacific Islander studies. *Applied Nursing Research* 24 (2): 9–15.

Liang CT, Li LC and Kim BS (2004) The Asian American racism-related stress inventory: development, factor analysis, reliability, and validity. *Journal of Counseling Psychology* 51 (1): 103–114.

Link BG and Phelan J (1995) Social conditions as fundamental causes of disease. *Journal of Health and Social Behavior* 35 (extra issue): 80–94.

Lyman SM (2000) The 'yellow peril' mystique: origins and vicissitudes of a racist discourse. *International Journal of Politics, Culture, and Society* 13 (4): 683–747.

McMurtry CL, Findling MG, Casey LS, Blendon RJ, Benson JM, Sayde JM and Miller C (2019) Discrimination in the United States: experiences of Asian Americans. *Health Services Research* 54 (S2): 1419–1430.

Molina N (2006) *Fit to be Citizens? Public Health and Race in Los Angeles, 1879–1939*. Los Angeles, CA: University of California Press.

Okamoto DG (2003) Toward a theory of panethnicity: explaining Asian American collective action. *American Sociological Review* 68 (6): 81–842.

Okamoto DG (2014) *Redefining Race: Asian American Panethnicity and Shifting Ethnic Boundaries*. New York: Russell Sage Foundation.

Omi M and Winant H (1994) *Racial Formation in the United States: From the 1960s to the 1990s*. New York: Routledge.

Paradies Y, Ben J, Denson N, Elias A, Priest N, Pieterse A, Gupta A, Kelaher M and Gee G (2015) Racism as a determinant of health: a systematic review and meta-analysis. *PloS One* 10 (9): e013851.

Paulose-Ram R, Burt V, Broitman L and Ahluwalia N (2017) Overview of Asian American data collection, release, and analysis: National Health and Nutrition Examination Survey 2011–2018. *American Journal of Public Health* 107 (6): 916–921.

Phelan JC and Link BG (2015) Is racism a fundamental cause of inequalities in health? *Annual Review of Sociology* 41: 311–330.

Ramakrishnan K, Junn J, Lee T and Wong J (2008) National Asian American Survey (NAAS), 2008. Retrieved from www.icpsr.umich.edu/web/RCMD/studies/31481 (accessed 2 October 2020).

Ramakrishnan, SK, Lee, J, Lee T and Wong J (2016) National Asian American Survey (NAAS) pre-election survey. Retrieved from www.icpsr.umich.edu/web/RCMD/studies/37024 (accessed 2 October 2020).

Ramakrishnan, SK, Lee J, Lee T and Wong J (2016) National Asian American Survey (NAAS) post-election survey. Retrieved from www.icpsr.umich.edu/web/RCMD/studies/37380 (accessed 2 October 2020).

Ruiz NG, Horowitz JM and Tamir C (2020) Many Black and Asian Americans say they have experienced discrimination amid the COVID-19 outbreak. Retrieved from www.pewsocialtrends.org/2020/07/01/many-black-and-asian-americans-say-they-have-experienced-discrimination-amid-the-covid-19-outbreak/ (accessed 2 October 2020).

Shah N (2001) *Contagious Divides: Epidemics and Race in San Francisco's Chinatown*. Los Angeles, CA: University of California Press.

Srinivasan S and Guillermo T (2000) Toward improved health: disaggregating Asian American and Native Hawaiian/Pacific Islander data. *American Journal of Public Health* 90 (11): 1731–1734.

Takaki R (1990) *Strangers from a Different Shore: A History of Asian Americans*. New York: Penguin Press.

Uehara ES, Takeuchi DT and Smukler M (1994) Effects of combining disparate groups in the analysis of ethnic differences: variations among Asian American mental health service consumers in level of community functioning. *American Journal of Community Psychology* 22 (1): 83–99.

United States Census Bureau (2020) 2018 American community survey 1-year estimate: Hispanic or Latino origin by race. Retrieved from https://data.census.gov/cedsci/table?q=race%20by%20hispanic&g=0100000US&tid=ACSDT1Y2018.B03002&hidePreview=false (accessed 6 October 2020).

Walton E (2009) Residential segregation and birth weight among racial and ethnic minorities in the United States. *Journal of Health and Social Behavior* 50 (4): 427–442.

Ward JW and Byrd KK (2012) Hepatitis B in the United States: a major health disparity affecting many foreign-born populations. *Hepatology* 56 (2): 419–421.

Xu J and Lee JC (2013) The marginalized 'model' minority: an empirical examination of the racial triangulation of Asian Americans. *Social Forces* 91 (4): 1363–1397.

Yan BW, Ng F, Chu Jet al. (2020) Asian Americans facing high COVID fatality. Retrieved from www.healthaffairs.org/do/10.1377/hblog20200708.894552/full (accessed 6 October 2020).

Yellow Horse AJ, Kuo K and Leong KJ. (2020) (eds) Viral racisms: Asians/Americans and Pacific Islanders respond to COVID-19. *Journal of Asian American Studies.*

Yoo HC, Gee GC and Takeuchi D (2009) Discrimination and health among Asian American immigrants: disentangling racial from language discrimination. *Social Science & Medicine* 68 (4): 726–732.

Zia H (2000) *Asian American Dreams: The Emergence of an American People*. New York: Farrar, Straus & Giroux.

17

AGEISM AND RISK DURING THE CORONAVIRUS PANDEMIC

Peta S. Cook, Cassie Curryer, Susan Banks, Barbara Barbosa Neves, Maho Omori, Annetta H. Mallon and Jack Lam

Introduction

The sudden risk and spread of the coronavirus, which was declared a global pandemic by the World Health Organization (2020) on 11 March 2020, has indelibly etched itself into social and public consciousness. Faced with the threat of COVID-19 infections and deaths, and the potential for the pandemic to place increasing burdens on healthcare systems, many countries have 'staged' precautionary safety measures to slow or contain the spread of the coronavirus. These measures included closing territorial borders, enforcing temporary closures on trading, hospitality and recreational venues, and introducing new policing and legal powers, including strict 'stay at home' measures and increased surveillance of social lives (Fernandes, 2020). These risk management or risk migration strategies regulate the activities of individuals, populations and economic systems. They involve risk discourses or frames that can cause 'othering' of specific behaviours or populations, which help shape public thinking about risk and vulnerability (McCormick and Whitney, 2013). Such discourses also fuel a range of discriminatory attitudes and actions towards certain individuals and populations (IFRC, UNICEF and World Health Organization, 2020), including stigma based on age.

In this chapter, we explore how the topic of COVID and age was framed or 'staged' in political and media discourses. Drawing on examples from Australian online media sources published in the early phase of the crisis (between March and April 2020), we shed light on how these risk discourses problematise and homogenise younger and older age groups as 'risky' and 'at risk', while also presenting confusing risk messages. To begin this discussion, we first explore some sociological perspectives on risk.

Understanding risk and the COVID pandemic sociologically

Sociologists locate risks in the social context. This context gives meaning to 'risk' and is – or becomes – connected to the actions of individuals, populations, and institutions. Within the 'world at risk' paradigm that builds on Ulrich Beck's risk society thesis, risks are '*future* events that *may* occur, that *threaten* us' (Beck, 2009: 9; emphasis added). This future focus means that risks are *anticipated* and *perceived*, conveying a sense of active control over the future. Regardless of whether the risks are real, imaginary or a social construction, they influence political decision-making as seen in strategies seeking to avert their occurrence. Risk calculations underpin these risk management strategies and policies in the hope of preventing, reducing or mitigating risk. As such, risk is viewed as undesirable, and framed as a hazard or danger that must be avoided. These institutionalised responses to risk scaffold it in a decision-making process and framework that assumes risks can be contained and controlled via policy or regulation.

Through the 'staging of risk' (Beck, 2009, 2011), which involves potential or projected future harms being produced through political and media discourses, institutional understandings of risk are represented and made publicly transparent. These risk representations operate as a form of power and social control, whereby 'some have the capacity to define risk and others do not' (Beck, 2009: 142). Such staging of risks is predominantly produced by institutional actors such as medical experts and politicians who are represented as acting in the public's (best) interests. While this process can help to create change (for example, increased public safety and preparedness), there are possibilities of misrepresentation and distortion, as well as an amplification of public anxieties, uncertainties and fears. Staging of risk can also lead to increasing surveillance of social life and reductions in individual freedoms, as witnessed by tighter airport security measures enacted in response to perceived terrorist threats in the past (Beck, 2009). During the coronavirus, this increasing surveillance of individuals is noticeable in smartphone COVID 'contact tracing' applications that draw on single or multiple technologies such as Bluetooth, geolocation data, data mining, and global position systems (GPS) (Howell O'Neill et al., 2020). Thus, the ways that risks are identified, staged, framed and communicated expose power relations and have important social and political implications (Abeysinghe and White, 2010; McCormick and Whitney, 2013).

The association between the staging of risk and the exercising of power can be seen in pandemic risk narratives that emerged from the zoonotic transmission of avian (H5N1) and swine (H1N1) influenza viruses into human populations. As noted by Abeysinghe and White (2010) and Fogarty et al. (2011), the dominant pandemic risk narratives in the media that emerged during the spread of H5N1 and H1N1, typically informed by government institutions and medical experts, may be used as a mechanism to gain political and economic advantages (Figuié, 2013). These pandemic frames include daily tallies of infection spread (for example, prevalence, incidence and mortality), pandemic preparedness (social, public, and individual), containment measures (such as testing, isolation and vaccine development) and, of interest in this chapter, the identification of groups considered to be 'vulnerable' (we are also interested in those cast as 'complacent').

These narratives that emerge from pandemic frames are often accompanied by increasing calls for calm, greater personal responsibility, exercising greater awareness of ones' own welfare and that of others, and public acceptance and engendering cooperation with measures aimed at managing risk and reducing the spread of disease (Fogarty et al., 2011). However, influenza control policies draw on a limited social imaginary of public responses that tend to frame the general publics as passive or vulnerable to the effects of pandemic influenza (Davis, Stephenson and Flowers, 2011). Under the 'virologic gaze' (Davis, Stephenson and Flowers, 2011: 916) of data gathering and epidemiological modelling, a key policy concern is how to ensure compliance with pandemic recommendations without invoking complacency or inciting panic in the general public. In the process, public health becomes conflated with national security and the identification and management of risk, as seen in the refusal of some countries to allow cruise ships from entering ports out of fear that passengers and crew might be infected with coronavirus (McCormick, 2020). Hence, the imposition of public health emergencies acts to reinforce public perceptions around pandemic risks and what constitutes 'risky' behaviour, allowing state and government authorities to assert social and technological control with minimal public feedback and indistinct (or unnamed) end-points (McCormick and Whitney, 2013). The experience of pandemic diseases is thus socially and politically constructed, as 'governments deploy technologies of risk to both frighten and motivate citizens' (Mythen and Walklate, 2008: 237). As a result, the information and advice presented in pandemic frames can be conflicting and lead to confusion and non-compliance.

Beck (2011: 1352) suggests that dealing with global risks drives an imperative to 'cooperate or fail' and therefore has the idealistic potential to include those populations who might normally experience social 'othering'. Yet the staging of risk could also amplify or create new forms of othering through the heightening of social fear and anxieties. For example, Douglas (1992, 2003) notes how perceptions of risk and danger are heavily informed by the social order, including socio-cultural norms and values. 'Others' can be blamed for risk, creating a dichotomy of 'us versus them' that confirms outsider and insider status. This process of 'othering', when applied by institutional actors, affirms social control and solidarity. As such, how risks are situated, framed and staged can benefit some at the expense of others (Beck, 2009).

Despite the institutionalisation of risk, individuals and populations can be made responsible for safeguarding (or surveilling) themselves and others, revealing that risk perceptions are also individual and relational. For example, during the enactment of the coronavirus physical distancing laws, Australian states and territories established online and telephone law enforcement hotlines to report non-compliance with quarantine or physical distancing restrictions, including violations of numerical limits for public or social gatherings (see, for example, Tasmania Police, 2020). Such rule of populations through state apparatuses facilitates population surveillance and interventions while reinforcing the need for individuals and populations to practise self-control and self-discipline (Foucault, 1998, 2003). As such, responsibility to manage institutional decisions and expert discourses (or responsibilisation) moves from the state to individuals, requiring the public to 'take responsibility' for themselves and others (Rose, 2000). This biopolitics relies on 'forecasts, statistical estimates, and overall measures' to manage and regulate individuals and populations, while punishing those engaging with undesirable conduct (Foucault, 2003: 246) During the coronavirus pandemic this included shaming people engaging in practices considered to be 'risky'.

Media perceptions are key to such processes, as they play a role in who are considered (in)capable and (un)able to take responsibility. Young et al. note that frequent media coverage of a disease:

> may influence the relationship between individuals' perceptions of population-level and individual-level risk. Individuals often exhibit 'unrealistic optimism', a disjuncture between their estimations of the risk to the general population which they are part of and their estimation of the same risk on a personal level.
>
> *(Young et al., 2013: 105)*

A more sinister outcome of media messages during the COVID crisis specifically has been the reproduction of a young/old risk assumption. This has clouded public health messages on viral spread, with physical distancing as being 'urgent' for older people but more unclear, fluid and relaxed for younger people. Such divisions between 'we' (or 'us') and 'them' replicate ageist ideas and values that separate younger and (in particular) older people from the rest of the population as 'special' or 'targeted' groups in their 'otherness'.

At the same time, individuals must self-manage the social traumas (as opposed to the biological consequences) of the coronavirus under a framework of solidarity – or in the words of Australian Prime Minister Scott Morrison (2020a), 'we'll get through this together Australia. We all have a role to play. Employers, nurses, doctors, teachers, scientists, friends, family and neighbours. I know we'll all do our bit'. However, such 'we are all in this together' rhetoric, associated with governing 'at a distance' (Dean, 2010; Foucault, 2003; Rose and Miller, 2010), ignores that some individuals and populations are more affected by COVID than others, and may also experience 'othering' through the political and media discourses and institutional responses to the coronavirus. This is evident when individuals or population groups are cast as a threat and danger; constructed as being 'at risk' or 'risky'. We now turn to these points.

Being 'at risk' and 'risky'

Within the context of influenza pandemics, Maunula (2013) conceives of individuals as 'pandemic subjects', and as medicalised and moral projects. Individuals are exhorted to willingly take up 'technologies of the self' in regulating their conduct

(Foucault, 1998) that, in the case of COVID, are witnessed in risk-minimisation behaviours. These include frequent handwashing, 'respiratory etiquette' (such as sneezing and coughing into one's elbow), self-monitoring of health, physical distancing and self-isolation. Those people who are perceived not to be complying with government recommendations for reducing and preventing the spread of infections are cast as immoral, irresponsible, and lacking self-control (Maunula, 2013). Within Australia and in the context of the coronavirus, the two population groups prominent in political and media discourses have been younger (adolescent, youth or young adults) and older (aged 70 years and over) people. The pandemic frames and staging of risk in media and political discourses focusing on these population groups have tended to differentiate them. This has typically involved framing younger people as 'risky' virus spreaders, and older people as 'at risk' from coronavirus. Paralleling this, another pandemic frame has younger people 'at risk' of a bleak economic future owing to coronavirus-related public health measures that are frequently framed as protecting 'the elderly' and 'the vulnerable'.

These dichotomous pandemic framings help to perpetuate generational divides while simultaneously diverting attention from discriminatory attitudes and practices, and from the wellbeing and health of the broader population. For example, the framing of older people as 'the elderly' or 'the vulnerable elderly' has reduced a large demographic – 15 per cent of Australia's total population in 2017 was 65 years of age or over (Australian Institute of Health and Welfare, 2018) – to a passive role. Words such as 'elderly' and 'seniors' are not neutral words; they are discriminatory and evoke a range of negative stereotypes that are often applied to older people as individuals and as a population (Lundebjerg et al., 2017). This can be seen in Australian critiques of political and public health responses to the coronavirus:

> *Many seniors* have had time to enjoy careers, children and grandchildren. My father is 68 and insists he's had a good run […] *Many seniors* like him would not put their own life above the livelihoods of their children and grandchildren, if the economic and social costs are too great. Yet [Australian Prime Minister] Morrison suggests people of all ages are equally worth saving.
>
> *(Kehoe, 2020; emphasis added)*

> […] we are asking the healthy, most of whom will be no more than inconvenienced by this latest strain of flu, to sacrifice or cripple themselves, their livelihoods, their children's future, to preserve people whose future is already precarious and limited. Has anyone checked with *the elderly*, who tend to have a more sanguine outlook, to see if this economic suicide is what they want?
>
> *(Waterson, 2020; emphasis added)*

In these examples, the economy is framed in relation to the capitalist labour market where workers earn wages from their labour while employers generate profit. While such understandings of economy can be critiqued, our interest is in how these comments demonstrate a process of 'othering'. The language – 'the elderly' and 'seniors' – segregates older people, separating them from other age groups and emphasising their alleged 'difference' (one of which is that they are deemed missing from the labour market or 'productive economy'). This reduces all people to *homo economicus*: motivated by their own self-interests to maintain wealth (or material wellbeing) and, within a capitalist framework, to maximise profits. As such, to let older people die is a way to 'reduce costs' and 'save the economy' from what Waterson (2020) labels as 'economic suicide', because older people are framed as 'unproductive'. Simultaneously, Kehoe (2020) and Waterson (2020) adopt a representative position, assigning specific traits and features to older people (for example, as grandparents or having a positive outlook) that homogenises older populations. In addition, Kehoe (2020) speaks *for* older people, rendering them voiceless and invisible.

This cultural script also negatively frames biological changes that *may* occur in later life: 'biological change is not necessarily decline' (Hepworth, 2003: 100). That is, a master social narrative of human ageing is reproduced, one that conflates older age with frailty, disability, redundancy, disengagement, being a 'burden' and decline (Gullette, 2018; Palmore, 2000). This is despite not all older people living with serious medical conditions or diseases, and over a third of Australians 75 years of age and over ranking their health as 'excellent/very good' (Australian Bureau of Statistics, 2019). While Australians are living longer and healthier lives (Goss, 2019), social attitudes regarding ageing often simplistically connect older age with decline (Gullette, 2018), as informed by social and medical normalisation of the 'youthful' body as the physiological, biological and aesthetic ideal. These discourses serve to limit the social and civic participation of older people, and mask, reduce or ignore the vast variability of their individual abilities and experiences. As such, chronological age is equated with social worth, which feeds oppression (Levy et al., 2014) and propagates ageism (prejudice and discrimination based on age).

Significantly, the comments made by Kehoe (2020) and Waterson (2020) further imply that older people are greedy and unless they accept they have 'had their turn' and express more concern regarding the economic future of the country and younger people, are responsible for the economic woes emerging from the public health and political responses to the coronavirus. Positioning older people as at fault insinuates that society is better off without older people and that they should 'die off' (Gullette, 2018: 259–260). In the case of the coronavirus, not expending resources on older people would be a benefit to the young, rather than seen as a loss of lives if older people happen to die. This perpetuates generational divisions and creates an artificial and misleading war between the health of the economy and the health (and lives) of older people. It is a zero-sum game: older people are framed as socially and economically worthless (and role-less) and unproductive (that is, not wage-earning) citizens. Within this pandemic framing, the value and worthiness of life is reductively measured in years.

The social privileging of youth, however, does not mean that younger people are immune from political and media scrutiny. In these pandemic framings, younger people have been cast as healthy, active, 'socially worthy' agents but also 'risky' by deliberately engaging in behaviours that risk their health and that of others. In Australia, a focus was placed on international backpackers staying in youth hostels as an example of the selfishness of younger people who prioritise their own self-interests over public health:

> We figure none of us have any symptoms, due to our age the virus is unlikely to get us, and we're more likely to get it in New York City where there are double the amount of cases than the 300 in Australia [...] I'm not nervous. I'm young. I feel my body can handle it.
>
> *(Young person quoted in Graham, 2020)*

Such reporting led to political condemnation of youth, with racist undertones: 'Those people with visas and backpackers have got to play by our rules, not by theirs' (Northern Beaches Local Councillor Pat Daley in Cross, 2020). Such critiques of the behaviours of younger people have contributed to the rise of the term 'Covidiot' – an individual who ignores public health and safety warnings or regulations or who hoards goods (for example, toilet paper) (see, Lawson, 2020). Constructing young people, including through selective reporting of 'covidiots' and infection naives (as in Graham, 2020, above) as risky rule-breakers is congruent with wider social stereotypes that younger people are unreliable, irresponsible, selfish, rebellious and requiring protection and disciplining as adults (or citizens) 'in training' (Bell, 2018; Ceaser, 2014). As such, these wilful risk takers pose a threat to collective social interests and values, requiring 'educating'.

These two groups, older and younger people, are linked by danger and threat, and by the staging of risk. Young people are carelessly risking the health of older people, and older people's vulnerability curbs economic activity to the detriment of the young. Both are subject to the shame and blame narratives that act to maintain social order. Risk is being used not only to reinforce desirable social behaviours but also, in the context of the coronavirus, to heighten awareness of danger (Douglas, 1992): danger to the economy and the danger of spreading coronavirus. Staging of risk justifies the unequal treatment of groups deemed dangerous such that 'a person has no place in the social system and is therefore a marginal being, all precaution against danger must come from others. He [sic] cannot help his abnormal situation' (Douglas, 2003: 98). Removing and marginalising are methods to protect others (and the economy) from danger associated with these age groups and their bodies.

Of course, this excludes those who are not deemed risky and are therefore not subject to the same framing. Arceneaux (2020) noted that 'The disease is spreading because the people in power – largely old white men – have failed the nation [the United States] by not properly preparing for its effects in spite of dire warnings'. Such critiques link to political and media narratives that downplayed the potential and real impacts of the coronavirus for those not considered not to be at risk. For example, Australian Prime Minister Morrison declared on 13 March 2020 that, as of 16 March 2020, non-essential mass gatherings of 500 people or more would be banned, but also proudly declared that he (one of the 'safe') would be attending a National Rugby League game on 14 March 2020; on which he later changed his mind after repeated questioning and pressure (Worthington, 2020). In his initial justification for attending, Morrison emphasised a staged and 'proportional' approach to risk management:

> These are stepped responses. We are not of any great concern right now in terms of where those gatherings might be today. But in the weeks ahead, in the weeks ahead, this will change. This is a matter of scaling our response [...] My point is there is, there is absolute reason for calm. There is absolute reason for proportionally responding to the challenges that we have here. [...] But right now, there is not that great risk. There is not that immediate threat. But these are things that will be scaled up in the weeks ahead.
>
> *(Morrison, 2020b)*

This is a fruitful example of the links between staging of risk and exercising power in pandemic responses – officials call for calm, while engaging in contradictory behaviour, messaging and selective risk awareness (Abeysinghe and White, 2010; Fogarty et al., 2011). Furthermore, as noted by Figuié (2013), risk can be deployed as a way of reinforcing political strength and its tactical management. The confusing messaging about the staging of risk, including who can do what and when, has impacts on how individuals and populations manage risk, and can cause uncertainty, confusion, and non-compliance.

Significantly, these confusing pandemic frames contrast infection-spread information with pandemic preparedness (or 'stepped responses'), while labelling risk groups such as 'the vulnerable elderly'. This is heightened through language use. For example, the pandemic framing 'only the elderly are at risk; young people don't have to worry' (Crescimanni, 2020) helps to cause misunderstanding about who is at risk. In addition, by stating 'only', little importance or relevance is attached to older people (thus reinforcing their unworthiness), and the potential consequences of the virus for the entire population are dismissed. As such, the response of 'I'm young. I feel my body can handle it' to the pandemic threat (young person quoted in Graham, 2020), can be viewed as a reflection of confusing media and political discourses, which includes differentiating between the perceived resilience of younger and older bodies. Such confusing messaging is also witnessed in the coronavirus being reduced to the 'latest strain of flu' (as seen previously in Waterson, 2020), and thus something familiar and a normal part of a yearly, seasonal cycle. In other words, official pandemic frames separate publics and rely on simplistic views of complacency and compliance, while also perpetuating ageist stereotypes and divisions.

Conclusion

The health and socioeconomic risks associated with the coronavirus are real and severe. However, these risks are amplified by their framing and the accompanying narrative. Those frames and narratives, based on one-dimensional understandings of complacency and compliance of publics, drive scenarios that justify heightening inequality and discrimination towards specific population groups. Some of these groups are more at risk of becoming ill from the coronavirus than others (for example, people with weakened immune systems or chronic medical conditions), but this risk cannot be simplistically reduced to age. That is, while the risks of moderate or severe illness, hospitalisation and death from COVID increase with age, it is the combination of older age with pre-existing health conditions such as one or more comorbidities (for example, hypertension and diabetes) and/or living in residential aged care home that increases susceptibility to and poor outcomes from COVID infection (Banerjee, D'Cruz and Sathyanarayana Rao, 2020; Perrotta et al. 2020). Chronological age *alone* is 'a very poor argument to determine an individual's usual state of health' (Rahman and Jahan, 2020), and is an unreliable indicator of someone's level or degree of vulnerability to COVID (Ehni and Wahl, 2020). Chronological age is also not an indicator of a person's abilities or social 'worth'.

These pandemic framings of COVID reinforce a social narrative wherein older persons are positioned as vulnerable and dependent and are therefore expendable, as self-management of risk is assigned as a capacity of young people alone – even when young people are framed as not necessarily behaving according to these scripts. These age-related scripts fail to capture the diversity and complexity of *all* age groups. Thus, it is important to acknowledge that how risks are framed results in differential experiences across and within different age groups.

In particular, we have shown in this chapter how this staging of risk and risk frames perpetuates ageism that positions young people as selfish risk takers in contrast to 'the vulnerable elderly' or 'frail elderly' who are at risk. This involves shaming and blaming based on age, with behaviours or traits stereotyped against certain age groups. These generational divides and dichotomous framings take a central role in how risk has been communicated during the coronavirus pandemic, with ageism and 'othering' shaping risk-management strategies and public messaging. It also leaves out a group of 'risk-free' people (presumably the 'middle-aged') from scrutiny or pandemic frames, as they are considered the norm and the default; neither 'vulnerable' nor 'reckless'. As risk perception is connected to health literacy and associated with the adoption of risk-reducing and protective behaviours, public health messages and measures can be undermined by complex, unclear, conflicting or false messaging (Dryhurst et al., 2020; Paakkari and Okan, 2020). Therefore, messaging about the staging of risk should not be nested in chronological age, as it can propagate ageism (Rahman and Jahan, 2020) and discrimination, present misleading representations of individuals and the COVID crisis, and cause confusion and uncertainty.

References

Abeysinghe S and White K (2010) Framing disease: the avian influenza pandemic in Australia. *Health Sociology Review* 19 (3): 369–381.

Arceneaux M (2020) Young people didn't social distance because the government kept telling them not to worry. *NBC News THINK*, 23 March. Retrieved from www.nbcnews.com/think/opinion/young-people-didn-t-social-distance-because-government-kept-telling-ncna1165281 (accessed 2 July 2020).

Australian Bureau of Statistics (2019) National health survey: first results, 2017–2018. Retrieved from www.abs.gov.au/AUSSTATS/abs@.nsf/Lookup/4364.0.55.001Main+Features100192017–18?OpenDocument (accessed 2 July 2020).

Australian Institute of Health and Welfare (2018) Older Australia at a glance. Retrieved from www.aihw.gov.au/reports-data/population-groups/older-people/overview (accessed 2 July 2020).

Banerjee D, D'Cruz MM and Sathyanarayana Rao TS (2020) Coronavirus disease 2019 and the elderly: focus on psychosocial well-being, agism, and abuse prevention – an advocacy review. *Journal of Geriatric Mental Health* 7 (1): 4–10.

Beck U (2009) *World at Risk*. Cambridge: Polity.

Beck U (2011) Cosmopolitanism as imagined communities of global risk. *American Behavioral Scientist* 55 (10): 1346–1361.

Bell J (2018) Adultism. In: Frey BB (ed.) *The Sage Encyclopedia of Educational Research, Measurement, and Evaluation*. Thousand Oaks, CA: Sage, pp. 55–57.

Ceaser D (2014) Unlearning adultism at Green Shoots: a reflexive ethnographic analysis of age inequality within an environmental education programme. *Ethnography and Education* 9 (2): 167–181.

Crescimanni TB (2020) I'm an Italian living in London. Barely any measures have been taken here against COVID-19 and we Italians are afraid. *Business Insider Italia*, 17 March. Retrieved from www.businessinsider.com/italian-london-covid-19-coronavirus-italians-afraid-2020-3?r=AU&IR=T (accessed 2 July 2020).

Cross J (2020) Northern Beaches Councillor Pat Daley: many backpackers should 'live by our rules'. *The Daily Telegraph*, 8 April. Retrieved from www.dailytelegraph.com.au/newslocal/manly-daily/northern-beaches-councillor-pat-daley-manly-backpackers-should-live-by-our-rules/news-story/8985879d96f32e6201965b8b4535202f (accessed 2 July 2020).

Davis M, Stephenson N and Flowers P (2011) Compliant, complacent or panicked? Investigating the problematisation of the Australian general public in pandemic influenza control. *Social Science & Medicine* 72 (6): 912–918.

Dean M (2010) *Governmentality: Power and Rule in Modern Society* (2nd ed.). London: Sage.

Douglas M (1992) *Risk and Blame: Essays in Cultural Theory*. London: Routledge.

Douglas M (2003) *Purity and Danger*. London: Routledge.

Dryhurst S, Schneider CR, Kerr J, Freeman ALJ, Recchia G, van der Bles AM, Spiegelhalter D and van der Linden S (2020) Risk perceptions of COVID-19 around the world. *Journal of Risk Research* 23 (7–8): 994–1006.

Ehni H-J and Wahl H-W (2020) Six propositions against ageism in the COVID-19 pandemic. *Journal of Aging & Social Policy* 32 (4–5): 515–525.

Fernandes A (2020) Electronic tracking devices among new coronavirus powers for WA security agencies. *SBS News*, 11 April. Retrieved from www.sbs.com.au/news/electronic-tracking-devices-among-new-coronavirus-powers-for-wa-security-agencies (accessed 30 June 2020).

Figuié M (2013) Global health risks and cosmopolitisation: from emergence to interference. *Sociology of Health & Illness* 35 (2): 227–240.

Fogarty AS, Holland K, Imison M, Blood RW, Chapman S and Holding S (2011) Communicating uncertainty how Australian television reported H1N1 risk in 2009: a content analysis. *BMC Public Health* 11 (1). Retrieved from https://bmcpublichealth.biomedcentral.com/articles/10.1186/1471-2458-11-181 (accessed 14 January 2021).

Foucault M (1988) Technologies of the self. In: Martin LH, Gutman H and Hutton PH (eds) *Technologies of the Self: A Seminar with Michel Foucault*. Amherst, MA: University of Massachusetts Press, pp. 16–49.

Foucault M (1998) *The Will to Knowledge: The History of Sexuality*, volume 1. London: Penguin.

Foucault M (2003) *Society Must be Defended: Lectures at the College de France, 1975–76*. London: Allen Lane.

Goss J (2019) We're not just living for longer – we're staying healthier for longer, too. *The Conversation*, 13 June. Retrieved from https://theconversation.com/were-not-just-living-for-longer-were-staying-healthier-for-longer-too-118588 (accessed 30 June 2020).

Graham B (2020) 'I'm young. I feel my body can handle it': Tourists ignore social distancing plea. *news.com.au*, 20 March. Retrieved from www.news.com.au/travel/travel-updates/im-young-i-feel-my-body-can-handle-it-tourists-ignore-social-distancing-plea/news-story/06221080d679aae68232fc9858de4f3f (accessed 30 June 2020).

Gullette MM (2018) Against 'aging' – how to talk about growing older. *Theory, Culture & Society* 35 (7–8):251–270.

Hepworth M (2003) Ageing bodies: aged by culture. In: Coupland J and Gwyn R (eds) *Discourse, the Body, and Identity*. London: Palgrave Macmillan, pp. 89–106.

Howell O'Neill P, Ryan-Mosely T and Johnson B (2020) A flood of coronavirus apps are tracking us. Now it's time to keep track of them. *MIT Technology Review*, 7 May. Retrieved from www.technologyreview.com/2020/05/07/1000961/launching-mittr-covid-tracing-tracker/ (accessed 12 June 2020).

IFRC, UNICEF and World Health Organization (2020) Social stigma associated with COVID-19. 24 February. Retrieved from www.who.int/docs/default-source/coronaviruse/covid19-stigma-guide.pdf (accessed 1 July 2020).

Kehoe J (2020) Lives matter but at what cost? *Financial Review*, 9 April. Retrieved from www.afr.com/politics/federal/lives-matter-but-at-what-cost-20200407-p54hox (accessed 30 June 2020).

Lawson R (2020) Coronavirus has led to an explosion of new words and phrases – and that helps us cope. *The Conversation*, 28 April. Retrieved from https://theconversation.com/coronavirus-has-led-to-an-explosion-of-new-words-and-phrases-and-that-helps-us-cope-136909 (accessed 30 June 2020).

Levy BR, Chung PH, Bedford T and Navrazhina K (2014) Facebook as a site for negative age stereotypes. *The Gerontologist* 54 (2): 172–176.

Lundebjerg NE, Trucil DE, Hammond EC and Applegate WB (2017) When it comes to older adults, language matters: 'Journal of the American Geriatrics Society' adopts modified American Medical Association style. *Journal of the American Geriatrics Society* 65 (7): 1386–1388.

McCormick E (2020) 'Stranded at sea': cruise ships around the world are adrift as ports turn them away. *The Guardian*, 27 March. Retrieved from www.theguardian.com/world/2020/mar/27/stranded-at-sea-cruise-ships-around-the-world-are-adrift-as-ports-turn-them-away (accessed 30 June 2020).

McCormick S and Whitney K (2013) The making of public health emergencies: West Nile virus in New York City. *Sociology of Health & Illness* 35 (2): 268–279.

Maunula L (2013) The pandemic subject: Canadian pandemic plans and communicating with the public about an influenza pandemic. *Healthcare Policy* 9: 14–25.

Morrison S (2020a) Address to the nation. 12 March. Retrieved from www.pm.gov.au/media/address-nation (accessed 30 June 2020).

Morrison S (2020b) Press conference with Premiers and Chief Ministers – Parramatta, NSW. 13 March. Retrieved from www.pm.gov.au/media/press-conference-premiers-and-chief-ministers-parramatta-nsw (accessed 30 June 2020).

Mythen G and Walklate S (2008) Terrorism, risk and international security: the perils of asking 'what if?'. *Security Dialogue* 39 (2–3): 221–242.

Paakkari L and Okan O (2020) COVID-19: health literacy is an underestimated problem. *The Lancet Public Health* 5 (5): e249–e250.

Palmore E (2000) Guest editorial: Ageism in gerontological language, *The Gerontologist* 40 (6): 645.

Perrotta F, Corbi1 G, Mazzeo G, Boccia M, Aronne L, D'Agnano V, Komici1 K, Mazzarella G, Parrella R and Bianco A (2020) COVID-19 and the elderly: insights into pathogenesis and clinical decision-making. *Aging Clinical and Experimental Research* 32. Retrieved from https://link.springer.com/article/10.1007/s40520-020-01631-y (accessed 14 January 2021).

Rahman A and Jahan Y (2020) Defining a 'risk group' and ageism in the era of COVID-19. *Journal of Loss and Trauma* 25 (8): 631–634.

Rose N (2000) Government and control. *The British Journal of Sociology* 40 (2): 321–339.

Rose N and Miller P (2010) Political power beyond the State: problematics of government. *The British Journal of Sociology* 61 (s1): 271–303.

Tasmania Police (2020) Tasmanian health hotline – form for reporting non-compliance. 7 May. Retrieved from www.police.tas.gov.au/services-online/tasmanian-health-hotline-form-for-reporting-non-compliance/ (accessed 27 June 2020).

Waterson S (2020) The analysis that divided Australia: join the debate. *The Australian*, 3 April. Retrieved from www.theaustralian.com.au/inquirer/national-coronavirus-hysteria-will-lead-to-disproportionate-suffering/news-story/56f887b32023c30efcc5f51346c92051 (accessed 30 June 2020).

World Health Organization (2020) WHO Director General's opening remarks at the media briefing on COVID-19. 11 March. Retrieved from www.who.int/dg/speeches/detail/who-director-general-s-opening-remarks-at-the-media-briefing-on-covid-19%2D%2D-11-march-2020 (accessed 30 June 2020).

Worthington B (2020) Gatherings of more than 500 people to be cancelled, Australians urged not to travel overseas amid coronavirus fears. *ABC News*, 14 March. Retrieved from www.abc.net.au/news/2020-03-13/coronavirus-scott-morrison-coag-premiers-cancelling-events/12053382 (accessed 30 June 2020).

Young ME, King N, Harper S and Humphreys KR (2013) The influence of popular media on perceptions of personal and population risk in possible disease outbreaks. *Health, Risk and Society* 15 (1): 103–114.

INDEX

Page numbers in **bold** refer to figures.

FSC
www.fsc.org
MIX
Papier | Fördert gute Waldnutzung
FSC® C083411

Kolibri 360 GmbH
Ferdinand-Jühlke-Straße 7
99095 Erfurt, Deutschland
produktsicherheit@kolibri360.de